Echocardiography in Adult Congenital Heart Disease

Wei Li, Michael Henein, and Michael A. Gatzoulis

Echocardiography in Adult Congenital Heart Disease

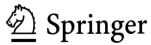 Springer

Wei Li, MD, PhD, FESC, FACC
Michael Henein, MSc, PhD, FESC, FACC, FAHA
Michael A. Gatzoulis, MD, PhD, FESC, FACC

Royal Brompton & Harefield NHS Trust
Imperial College School of Medicine
London
UK

British Library Cataloguing in Publication Data
Li, Wei
    Echocardiography in adult congenital heart disease
    1. Congenital heart disease—Diagnosis   2. Echocardiography
    I. Title   II. Henein, Michael Y., 1959–   III. Gatzoulis,
    Michael A.
    616.1′2′043
ISBN-13: 9781846288159

Library of Congress Control Number: 2007921870

ISBN: 978-1-84628-815-9   e-ISBN: 978-1-84628-816-6

Printed on acid-free paper

© Springer-Verlag London Limited 2007

9 8 7 6 5 4 3 2 1

Springer Science+Business Media
springer.com

Foreword

Due to the success of surgical repair of congenital cardiac defects, the population of adults with congenital heart defects is increasing rapidly. In fact, it is estimated that there are now more adults than children with congenital heart disease in the United States. Although surgical repair is now relatively safe and survival into adulthood is assured for the majority of infants born with congenital heart disease, such individuals are not "cured" and usually have a variety of residua and sequelae of the original defect and the surgical repair. Late complications are common and life expectancy remains limited for a large number of these patients.

With an increasing population and persistent clinical problems, it is inevitable that these patients require ongoing cardiac care throughout their lifetimes. Despite the fact that some regional centers of excellence for the care of the adult with congenital heart disease exist, many such patients present in community hospital and primary care settings.

Echocardiography is the definitive imaging tool for evaluation of infants and children with congenital heart disease, and remains the staring point for initial evaluation of the adult with congenital heart disease. In conjunction with a physical examination and a complete history, including initial diagnosis and subsequent surgical interventions, an echocardiographic examination is essential in the evaluation of any patient with congenital heart disease. However the professional who performs the echocardiographic study and the physician who interprets the images must understand the terminology of congenital heart disease and recognize the characteristic images and flow patterns associated with the various lesions encountered in this patient population.

Drs. Li, Henein, and Gatzoulis are internationally renown experts from the Royal Brompton National Heart and Lung Hospital, arguably the premier adult congenital cardiac center in the world. They have produced a volume that is neither an encyclopedic compendium nor a massive echocardiographic atlas. It is, rather, a thorough overview of the important aspects of echocardiographic evaluation of adults with congenital heart disease. Nearly every page contains echo images illustrating various views and findings for each type of congenital defect. Echocardiography critically influences patient management and this book puts the echo findings into an appropriate clinical perspective. The authors have also included information from other imaging modalities, such as MRI, which serve as reminders of the complementary role of various techniques in the evaluation and management of this complex patient population.

Echocardiography in Adult Congenital Heart Disease is an indispensable reference for anyone involved in imaging patients with congenital heart defects. It will introduce some readers to the subject of adult congenital heart disease and serve as a refresher for others. I hope that it will engage you and encourage you to read more, seek out original sources and increase your knowledge of this important field. This book will serve each of us in our role as lifelong learners and compel us to answer questions, produce new knowledge and teach others.

Daniel J. Murphy, Jr., MD
Stanford, California
May 2007

Preface

Doppler echocardiography has become the mainstay of adult cardiology practice worldwide. It provides essential information on cardiac anatomy and physiology. Its ease of use and complementary role to the bed-side examination has even given it he name of the "imaging stethoscope."

In *Echocardiography in Adult Congenital Heart Disease,* we present our clinical experience in applying echocardiographic techniques specifically to the diagnosis and management of adult patients with congenital heart disease. Wherever possible, we have tried to provide suggestions for the adaptation of standard imaging protocols to accommodate specific congenital heart conditions. The extremely varied morphologic spectrum of congenital heart disease, however, reinforces the need for describing individual components of anatomy, that is, the atrioventricular and ventriculoarterial connections, and this cannot be overemphasized for complex lesions.

Our practical textbook provides an anatomical basis for these malformed hearts, together with a discussion of the physiological patterns seen in different conditions. Our focus has been on contemporary clinical practice. We have, thus, related imaging to the clinical status of the patient, and provided information on disease progression and the effects of further intervention whether surgical or catheter.

We hope that we have given a sufficient number of examples of the many different conditions and variations on physiology to have written a useful guide for the diagnosis and management of your patients with congenital heart disease We have made this book a focused manual, which can be kept by the echo machine for easy reference, rather than a large textbook, which might gather dust on a shelf. This means that we have, to some extent, sacrificed additional information, which would have had less impact on day-to-day practice and would have made it more difficult to follow. We have also used terminology and descriptions with which both paediatric and adult congenital heart disease practitioners will be acquainted.

We are indebted to our patients who gave us such an opportunity to improve our understanding of congenital heart disease; clearly, without them this book would not have been possible.

We would value a great deal your feedback as to what else you would like to see included in the second edition and any comments on how we can make this focused textbook better for your day-to-day echocardiographic practice.

Wei Li
Michael Henein
Michael A. Gatzoulis
London, UK

Contents

1
Septal Defects

1.1. Interatrial Communication

Atrial septal defect is one of the most common lesions in adult congenital cardiac anomalies. It is characterized by the defects occurring in structures that separate the two atria, and thus permit shunting of blood from the high pressure atrium to the low pressure atrium. Patients may remain asymptomatic during the first few decades of life. Most patients are accidentally diagnosed in cardiology clinics after presenting with a heart murmur incidently, and fixed split second heart sound, right bundle branch block on ECG or signs of right heart dilatation on chest X-ray or transthoracic echocardiography. Later an exertional and dyspnea, atrial arrhythmia may become the common presentation that guides diagnosis.

Atrial septal defects are classified into six different types according to their anatomical location: secundum (oval fossa), primum (partial atrioventricular septal defect), superior sinus venosus, inferior sinus venosus, coronary sinus, and confluent or common atrium type.

1.1.1. Secundum Atrial Septal Defect

This is the most common form of atrial septal defect. The defect is located either at the fossa ovale or adjacent region. The size of the defect varies from very small (patent foramen ovale) to a large one that may exceed 4 cm in diameter. Large defects may extend to involve the upper region of the atrial septum close to the superior vena caval orifice. Very small defects (small patent foramen ovale) may be associated with intermittent left-to-right shunt compared with the continuous left-to-right shunt that is commonly seen in good-sized defects, unless very significant right ventricular and/or increased right atrial pressure are present. With diastolic dysfunction shunt direction may be right to left.

1.1.1.1. Echocardiography

A modified apical four chamber view (from conventional four chamber view, move the probe towards the sternum until the atrial septum is nearly

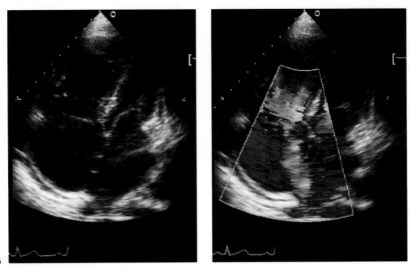

FIGURE 1.1. (A) A modified four chamber view showing an echo dropout at the mid-atrial septum. (B) Color flow Doppler from the same patient showing left-to-right shunt across the defect.

perpendicular to the ultrasound beam and then angulate anteriorly) is the best view to study the atrial septum with fine adjustments. An echo dropout at the middle portion of the atrial septum with well-defined edges suggests the presence of atrial septal defect. Color flow Doppler confirms the anatomical diagnosis and the shunt but on its own may mask the presence of left-to-right shunt in patients with raised right atrial pressure (see Figure 1.1).

Subcostal view with the echo beam perpendicular to the atrial septum may be helpful in diagnosing small shunts in adult patients that are difficult to be seen from the parasternal window. Unlike in children, subcostal images in adults may provide unsatisfactory image quality (see Figure 1.2).

1.1.1.1.1. Atrial Septal Defect

1.1.1.1.1.1. Size Assessment. An atrial septal defect should not be assumed to be always circular in shape, therefore measurements should be made from different views and the largest diameter should be considered for management and decision making. The defect diameter is measured from the two edges seen on the two-dimensional images. If the edges are not clearly seen the diameter is measured from a frozen image of the color Doppler jet across the septal defect. Presently developed real-time three-dimensional echocardiography provides a unique tool for assessing the shape and overall diameter of the

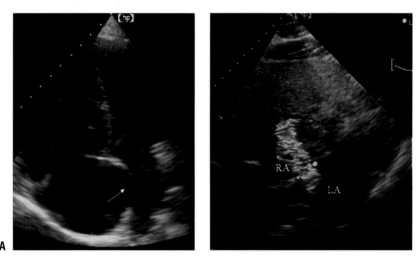

Figure 1.2. (A) Apical four chamber view demonstrating dilated right heart and possible secundum atrial septal defect (*arrow*). (B) Subcostal view showing an echo dropout at the mid-atrial septum and color flow Doppler showing left-to-right shunt.

atrial septal defect. It provides direct enface view of the septal defect from the atrium, particularly in sizable defects, that guides operators to the best decision making and management. Three-dimensional color flow measurements may improve the accuracy of shunt quantification (see Figures 1.3 and 1.4).

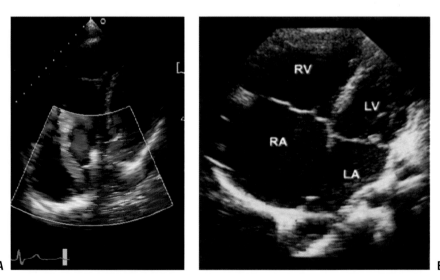

Figure 1.3. (A) Color flow Doppler (modified apical four chamber view) from a patient with a small atrial septal defect (narrow jet) 5 mm in diameter. (B) Similar images from a patient with a large atrial septal defect showing a defect diameter of 30 mm.

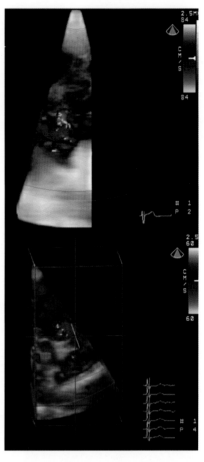

FIGURE 1.4. (A) Real-time three-dimensional images from a patient with large atrial septal defect, an enface view from the left atrium. (B) Similar images with color flow Doppler across the defect.

1.1.1.1.1.2. Shunt Quantification. Shunt quantification can be made from the difference between left and right ventricular estimated cardiac output. This is based on the assessment of stroke volume from the velocity time integral of the aortic and pulmonary flow velocities multiplied by respective outflow tract cross sectional area. Shunt ratio above 1.5 is usually considered significant enough to warrant closure (see Figure 1.5).

1.1.1.1.1.3. Complications of Longstanding Atrial Septal Defect.
Right Heart Dilatation. In patients with small atrial septal derfect, the right heart may be completely normal in size and function. However, a moderate-sized atrial septal defect is usually associated with a significant right atrial and right

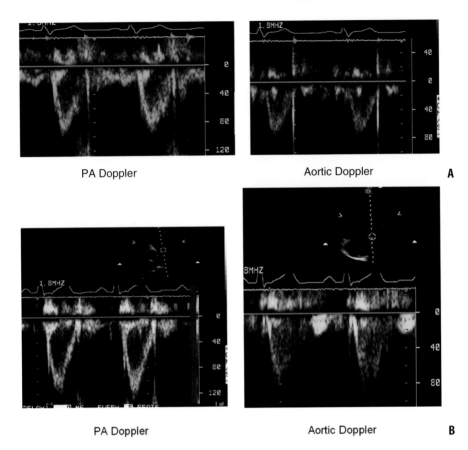

PA Doppler   Aortic Doppler   **A**

PA Doppler   Aortic Doppler   **B**

FIGURE 1.5. Velocity time integral (VTI) of the pulmonary and aortic flow from two patients with atrial septal defect, showing a small shunt in one patient (A) and large shunt in another (B). Note the significant difference in VTI ratio between the two patients.

ventricular dilatation, unless the right ventricle is physiologically restrictive (stiff) or hypoplastic.

Increased pulmonary flow velocities and velocity time integral (VTI) usually represent a large left-to-right shunt. Velocities may exceed 3 to 4 m/s (reflecting a physiologically narrowed pulmonary valve area). Although these velocities are functional in origin, a mild degree of organic pulmonary stenosis may also coexist with atrial septal defects. The main pulmonary artery and branches may also be markedly dilated in some patients (see Figure 1.6–1.8).

Tricuspid Regurgitation. In the absence of tricuspid valve disease, tricuspid regurgitation in patients with atrial septal defect is usually mild in severity. In elderly patients with longstanding severe right ventricular overload that results

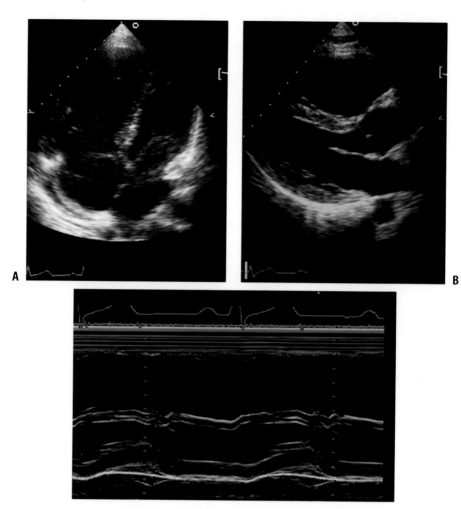

FIGURE 1.6. (A) Apical and (B) parasternal views showing right atrial and ventricular dilatation from a patient with atrial septal defect.

in tricuspid ring dilatation, a moderate degree of tricuspid regurgitation may be seen (see Figure 1.9).

Pulmonary Arterial Hypertension. Pulmonary arterial hypertension develops with advancing age in patients with atrial septal defect. It is well known that pulmonary artery pressure increases by 10 mm Hg per decade. Severe pulmonary hypertension is a rare complication; however, with shunt reversal Eisenmenger additional pathology should be sought (e.g., thromboembolic disease). The severity of pulmonary arterial hypertension can be estimated from the continuous wave Doppler velocities of the tricuspid and pulmonary valves; peak pulmonary artery pressure from tricuspid regurgitation velocity

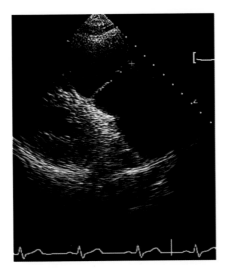

FIGURE 1.7. Parasternal short-axis view from the same patient showing dilated main pulmonary artery.

and mean pressure from the pulmonary regurgitation velocities. The modified Bernoulli equation, $PAP = 4V^2 + RA$ pressure, is used, where PAP is pulmonary artery pressure, V is the peak retrograde blood velocity across tricuspid and the pulmonary valves, and RA is estimated right atrial pressure. Underestimation of right atrial pressure may overestimate the peak pulmonary artery pressure (see Figure 1.10), based on pressure difference between the right ventricle and the right atrium.

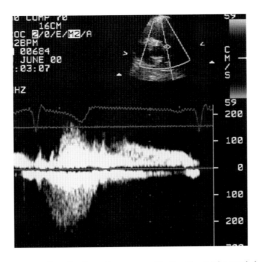

FIGURE 1.8. Continuous wave Doppler from the same patient with atrial septal defect showing raised forward pulmonary velocities of 2.5 m/s (secondary to increased right ventricular stroke volume).

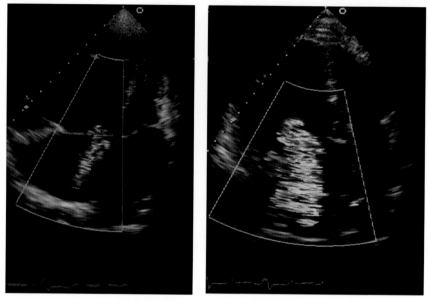

A   **B**

FIGURE 1.9. (A) Apical four chamber view from a patient with mild tricuspid regurgitation on color flow Doppler and (B) from a patient with a large right heart and moderate tricuspid regurgitation.

1.1.2. Primum Atrial Septal Defect

Primum atrial septal defect is also called partial atrio ventricular septal defect. This type of defect is located at the bottom of the atrial septum with the two atrioventricular (AV) valves at the same level. The left AV valve is trileaflet; left AV valve regurgitation is a common finding in this lesion. Valve regurgitation

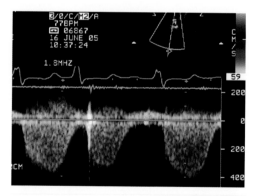

FIGURE 1.10. Continuous wave Doppler of tricuspid regurgitation from a patient with atrial septal defect showing signs of raised pulmonary artery pressure; peak pressure difference of 60 mm Hg between right ventricle (RV) and right atrium (RA).

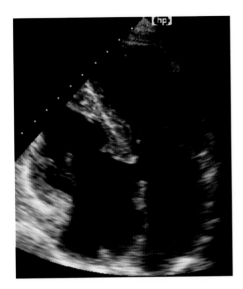 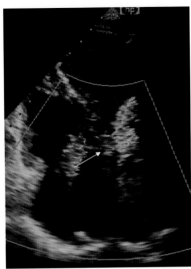

FIGURE **1.11.** Transthoracic apical four chamber view from a patient with a primum atrial septal defect showing complete absence of septal tissue at the region of the central fibrous body.

usually originates from the superior commissure of the valve. As a result of the left AV valve abnormality, the shorter inlet to outlet camponent of the left ventricle and the unwedged position of the aorta the left ventricular outflow tract becomes elongated (goose neck deformity) and may become stenotic. Left AV valve regurgitation contributes significantly to the left atrial dilatation known in this condition (see Figures 1.11 and 1.12).

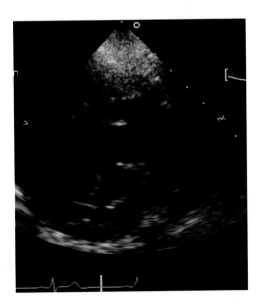

FIGURE **1.12.** Transthoracic parasternal short axis view showing trileaflet left AV valve.

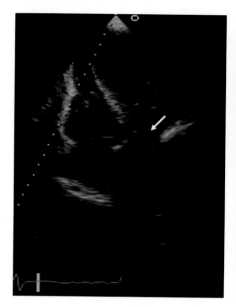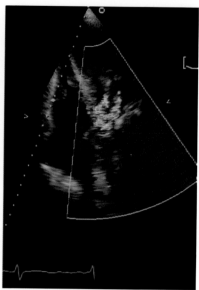

FIGURE 1.13. Apical five chamber view from a patient with repaired primum atrial septal defect showing narrowed left ventricular outflow tract (*arrow*).

Management of primum atrial septal defect is surgical closure. Surgical closure of such a defect may result in left ventricular outflow tract narrowing and, consequently, high pressure gradient, particularly with fast heart rate (see Figure 1.13). Late development of complete heart block is another late complication that needs regular follow up.

Left AV valve regurgitation tends to worsen with time in such patients; therefore, may require further repair or occasionally valve replacement (see Figure 1.14).

1.1.3. Superior Vena Cava Defect

Sinus venous defects are easily missed by transthoracic echocardiography. The defect is bordered either by the superior vena cava, the inferior vena cava, or the coronary sinus. Superior vena cava atrial septal defect is the most common type. Modified parasternal transthoracic echocardiographic views are the most helpful in diagnosing such defect in most cases. Sinus venosus defects are often associated with anomalous pulmonary venous drainage. When it occurs it adds to the volume overload of the right ventricle, thus resulting in disproportionate right heart dilatation with respect to the atrial septal defect diameter.

Even in the absence of a clear evidence for direct shunt, right heart chamber dilatation warrants further investigation to ascertain exclusion of this rare type of defect. Furthermore, disproportionate dilatation of the right heart in the

Before   After

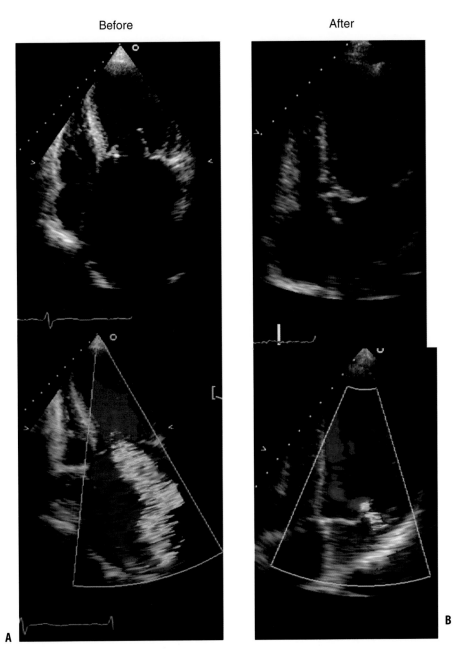

A   B

FIGURE 1.14. Severe left-side atrioventricular valve regurgitation before (A) and after (B) primum atrial septal defect repair.

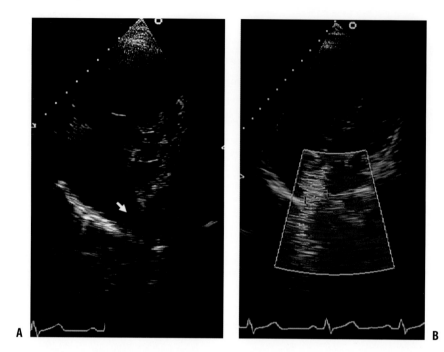

FIGURE **1.15.** (A) Modified parasternal five chamber view from a patient with sinus venosus atrial septal defect; note the echo dropout at the top of the atrial septum. (B) Left-to-right shunt on color Doppler.

presence of a relatively small sinus venosus defect suggests the possibility of coexisting anomalous pulmonary venous drainage. Transesophageal echocardiography adds more certainty to the final diagnosis of associated anomalies (see Figures 1.15 and 1.16).

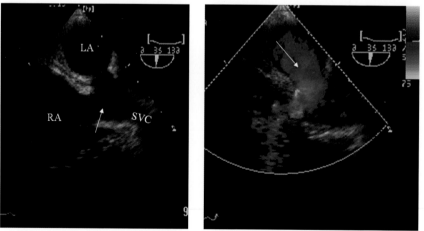

FIGURE **1.16.** (A) Transesophageal echocardiogram from a patient with a superior vena cava (*arrow*) atrial septal defect and (B) color flow Doppler showing left-to-right shunt across the defect.

1.1.4. Inferior Vena Cava Defect

This type of defect is less common than the superior vena cava defect. Inferior vena caval lesion is best diagnosed from the subcostal view when demonstrating two vena cavae inlet to the right atrium or by transesophageal echocardiography. Patients with inferior vena cava defect may be cyanosed as a result of the overriding of the atrial septal defect by the inferior vena cava with right-to-left shunt.

1.1.5. Coronary Sinus Defect

Coronary sinus defect represents a deficiency of the wall between the coronary sinus and the left atrium (or partially unroofed coronary sinus). This type of defect is rare and is best seen from the apical four chamber view with a slight posterior angulation of the probe to image the coronary sinus or from subcostal parasagital view. The coronary sinus is often dilated and this lesion is usually associated with persistence of left superior caval vein. Like the inferior vena cava defect, patients with coronary sinus defect may be cyanosed as the venous blood from coronary sinus with left SVC drains into the left atrium. Transesophageal echocardiography provides clearer images of the defect (see Figure 1.17).

1.1.6. Confluent or Common Atrium

A large confluence defect between the two atria is often associated with other congenital malformations, such as partial anomalous pulmonary venous

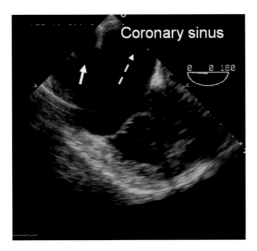

FIGURE 1.17. Transesophageal echocardiogram from a patient with coronary sinus defect; note coronary sinus is markedly dilated.

connection, persistent left-side SVC (superior vena cava), pulmonary valve stenosis or left atrial isomerism, etc. This is a very rare anomaly.

1.1.7. Management of Atrial Septal Defects

Atrial septal defects with evidence of right heart dilatation warrant elective closure irrespective of patient's age. The majority of secundum atrial septal defects can be closed by percutaneous devices. Suitability for device closure depends on detailed echocardiographic assessment and demonstration of sufficient (more than 5 mm) tissue edges around the defect. Large atrial septal defects of more than 40 mm in diameter may require surgical closure. Surgical closure or repair is the only choice for the other forms of atrial septal defects (see Figure 1.18).

1.1.7.1. Patent Foramen Ovale

In adult congenital heart disease clinics, diagnosis of patent foramen ovale has become an increasing clinical request due to its association with cerebrovascular accidents, strokes, and migraine. Patent foramen ovale (PFO) is a defect due to the flap valve of the oval fossa that fails to seal with the rim, which permits right-to-left shunt when the right atrial pressure is higher than that of the left. It sometimes allows left-to-right shunt. Although in most instances

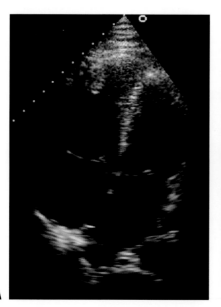
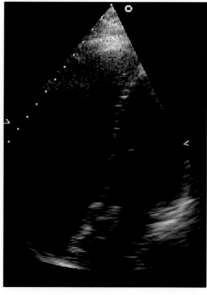

A   B

FIGURE 1.18. Apical four chamber view from a patient with secundum atrial septal defect (A) before and (B) after device closure.

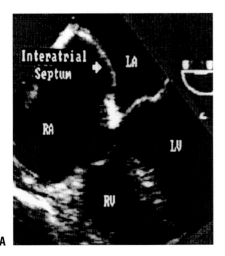
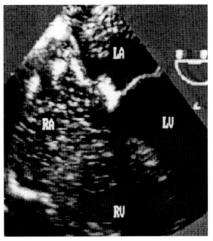

FIGURE 1.19. (A) Transesophageal echocardiogram of four chamber view from a patient with aneurysmal middle third of the interatral septum and (B) contrast injection demonstrating a right-to-left shunt with Valsalva manoeuvre.

there is a single defect, it is not unusual to identify additional fenestrations, often associated with an aneurysm of oval fossa. Contrast echocardiography with Valsalva maneuver is the most effective diagnostic tool for this condition. The timing and extent of right-to-left contrast shunt reflects the size of the defect (see Figures 1.19 to 1.21).

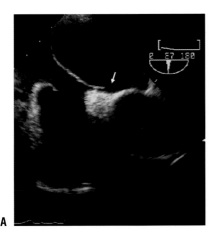
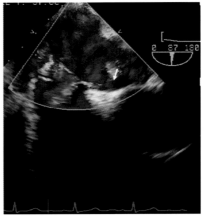

FIGURE 1.20. (A) Transesophageal echocardiogram showing a patent foramen ovale. (B) Color Doppler shows right-to-left shunt across a patent foramen ovale.

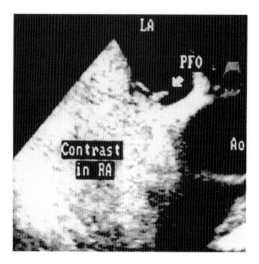

FIGURE 1.21. Transesophageal echocardiography contrast shows right-to-left shunting through a patent foramen ovale.

1.2. Ventricular Septal Defect

Ventricular septal defect represents discontinuity of the ventricular septum that results in left-to-right shunting.

1.2.1. Classification

1. **Perimembranous Ventricular Septal Defect.** This defect occupies the area of the membranous septum or part of its border that is anatomically formed by the fibrous continuity between the leaflets of atrioventricular valve and semilunal valve, tricuspid and aortic valve respectively in normal hearts. According to the location, these lesions can be described as subtricuspid or subaortic ventral septal defect. The defect can also extend so that it opens from the subaortic area into the inlet, outlet, or trabecular portions of the right ventricle, or they can be large and confluent.

2. **Muscular Ventricular Septal Defect.** This defect has muscular border and can be described as muscular inlet, outlet, or apical trabecular ventricular septal defect.

3. **Doubly Committed Subarterial Ventricular Septal Defect.** This type of defect is characterized by fibrous continuity between the adjacent leaflets of the aortic and pulmonary valves. Superiorly, these defects are roofed by arterial valves while posteroinferiorly the margin may be muscular or perimembranous.

Ventricular septal defects can be (1) small in size with no hemodynamic consequences, but they carry the risk of potential superimposed infection (endocarditis); (2) large in size, the majority of which develop pulmonary hypertension and with time reversal of shunt and cyanosis (Eisenmenger syndrome); or (3) residual defects after repair.

1.2.1.1. Echocardiography

Ventricular septal defects should be imaged from several planes in order to provide a precise diagnosis. Parasternal short-axis view is used to determine the exact site of the lesion. For the perimembranous ventricular septal defect, parasternal short-axis and apical four chamber views show the proximity of the defect to the tricuspid valve, while parasternal and apical long-axis views demonstrate the relationship of the defect to the aortic valve. Perimembranous ventricular septal defects extending to the inlet portion are best shown in the apical four chamber or subcostal paracoronal view. For apical trabecular muscular ventricular septal defect, parasternal short-axis view while scanning towards the apex demonstrates the left-to-right shunt on color flow Doppler. For doubly committed and juxta-arterial defects, the parasternal long-axis view with anterosuperior angulation or subcostal parasagittal planes can display the continuity of both arterial valves and also the presence, if any, of herniation of the right-facing aortic sinus. Residual ventricular septal defect postsurgical repair is often around the patch (see Figures 1.22 to 1.25).

1.2.2. Complications of Ventricular Septal Defect

1.2.2.1. Left Ventricular Dilatation and Dysfunction Associated with Small Defects

Small ventricular septal defects may be associated with some degree of left ventricular dilatation and, in adult patients, independent left ventricular

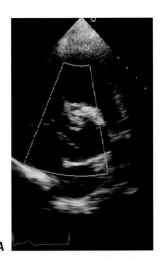
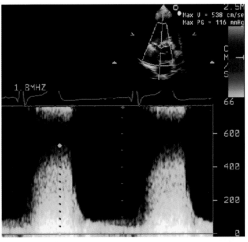

A   B

FIGURE 1.22. (A) Short-axis view from a patient with a perimembranous subtricuspid small ventricular septal defect and (B) continuous wave Doppler showing high velocity left-to-right shunting.

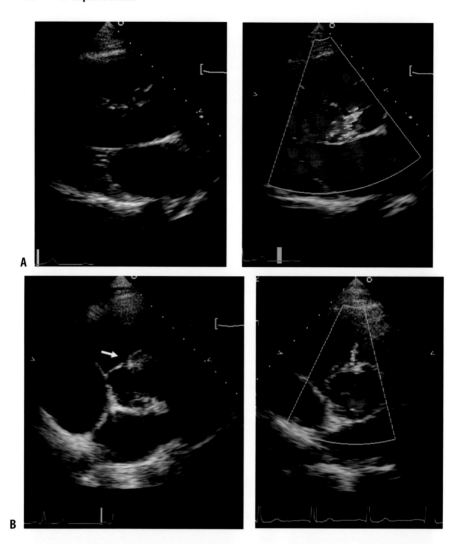

FIGURE 1.23. (A) Parasternal long-axis view and (B) corresponding short-axis images from a patient with a subaortic ventricular septal defect showing the defect at 12 o'clock. The long-axis view also shows the aortic cusps prolapsing into the VSD causing partial closure of the defect. Note the resulting mild aortic regurgitation on color Doppler.

systolic dysfunction may be present. With left ventricular dysfunction, left-to-right shunt through the defect occurs not only during systole but also during diastole. This results in increased shunt volume. The left-to-right shunt velocity during diastole also reflects the left ventricular end diastolic pressure (see Figure 1.26).

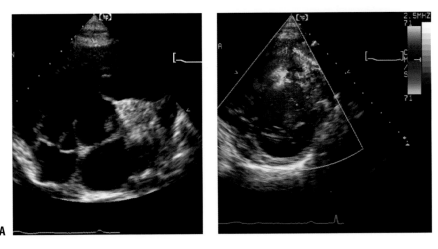

A   **B**

FIGURE 1.24. (A, B) Short-axis view from a patient with doubly committed ventricular septal defect and Eisenmenger syndrome showing a dilated right heart. Note key anatomical feature of such a defect the fibrous continuity between pulmonary and aortic valve.

1.2.2.2. Aortic Regurgitation

Because of the location of the subaortic defect, aortic leaflets may prolapse into the ventricular septal defect. This results in failure of the aortic leaflets to coapt, and, consequently, aortic regurgitation of various severity develops. With time

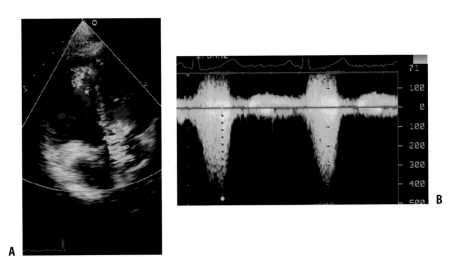

A   **B**

FIGURE 1.25. (A) Apical four chamber view showing a small apical muscular ventricular septal defect with left-to-right shunt on color flow and (B) continuous wave Doppler.

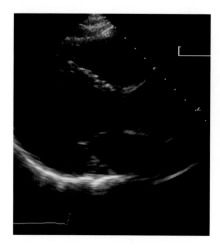
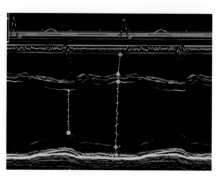

FIGURE 1.26. Parasternal views from a patient with a small ventricular septal defect showing dilated left ventricle on two-dimensional and M-mode images. Note the significant impairment of left ventricular systolic function, estimated fractional shortening of 20%. This patient's main complaint was syncope.

the ventricular septal defect may become progressively smaller in size while aortic regurgitation worsens in severity. Patients presenting with such picture may need surgical repair to guard against ventricular dysfunction caused by the severe aortic regurgitation (see Figure 1.27).

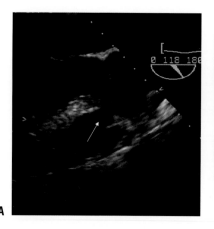
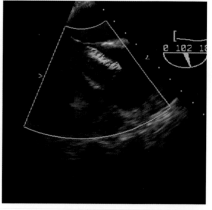

A

B

FIGURE 1.27. (A) Transesophageal echocardiogram of left ventricular outflow from a patient with subaortic ventricular septal defect and aortic regurgitation. Note the defect is just beneath the right coronary cusp. (B) The deformed aortic valve leads to aortic regurgitation.

1.2.3. Management

Hemodynamically significant ventricular septal defects need closure either surgically or by percutaneous device implantation. Decision making depends on the defect position and size. Echocardiography combining transthoracic and transesophageal provides accurate information on the exact location of the defect. The defect size is usually measured on the two-dimensional images from the leading edges or from color flow jet diameter. Disproportionate left ventricular dilatation in patients with modest defect size suggests the presence of additional shunt, which, if excluded, a diagnosis of dilated cardiomyopathy can be made. Shunt calculations are made in the same way as in the atrial septal defect from the left and right ventricular relative outflow tract velocity time–integral relationships.

1.2.4. Intraoperative Echocardiography

Transesophageal echocardiography or intracardiac echocardiography guides operators to the accurate position of the septal defect and the precise placement of the closure device. It also assists in excluding any significant additional lesion that might have been overlooked by the preoperative transthoracic echocardiographic assessment. During surgical repair transesophageal echocardiography confirms complete sealing of the defect and excludes any residual shunt.

Subacute bacterial endocarditis and Eisenminger physiology will be discussed in separate chapters.

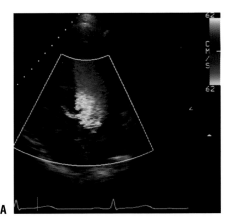
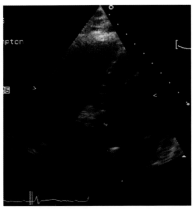

A   B

FIGURE 1.28. Apical four chamber view from a patient with a perimembranous ventricular septal defect (A) before and (B) after device closure of the defect. Note the device position that resulted in complete sealing of the defect.

1.3. Atrioventricular Septal Defects

Atrioventricular septal (canal) defect occurs at the atrioventricular junction (top end of the ventricular septum and bottom end of the inter atrial septum). Atrioventricular septal defects represent a spectrum of lesions with a potential for shunting at the atrial level as exemplified by ostium primum defects or at the ventricular level or at both levels. The size of the defect is variable as is the arrangement of the valvar leaflets with respect to each other and to the septum. When the ventricular septal defect is large, pulmonary hypertension develops early in life. Patients with small defects may remain asymptomatic for a long time. Atrioventricular septal defect is commonly seen in patients with Down syndrome.

In adult population, the following groups of patients are seen:

- Partial atrioventricular septal defect or primum atrial septal defect or atrio-ventricular septal defect with small ventricular component with no or mild-to-moderate pulmonary hypertension. Such patients have two separate AV valves.
- Large complete atrioventricular septal defect and a single common AV valve with established Eisenmenger physiology, often associated with Down syndrome.
- Repaired atrioventricular septal defect (including primum strial septal defect). The majority of patients after surgical repair have good hemodynamic results and remain asymptomatic. Some patients may have residual shunt, left or right atrioventricular valve regurgitation, or left ventricular outflow tract obstruction. In rare cases, pulmonary hypertension progresses despite the repair of the shunt. Atrioventricular valve stenosis is rarely seen after repair. All patients with atrioventricular septal defect are predisposed to complete heart block irrespective of surgery.

1.3.1. Echocardiography

The commonly used view to establish the diagnosis of atrioventricluar septal defect is the parasternal long-axis view, which demonstrates the elongated left ventricular outflow tract (the characteristic gooseneck deformity) and the abnormal trileaflets left atrioventricular valve with septal attachment. Apical four chamber view is the preferred diagnostic image that displays the loss of the offset arrangement of left and right atrioventricular valve leaflets. Anterior angulation of the transducer displays the anterosuperior bridging leaflet. Parasternal short-axis view demonstrates five leaflet arrangement of the common atrioventricular valve and the trileaflet left component. In adults with atrioventricular septal defect, either the left or the right atrioventricular valve may be incompetent and result in significant clinical consequences. Significant left ventricular outflow tract obstruction may develop later after surgical repair (see Figure 1.29).

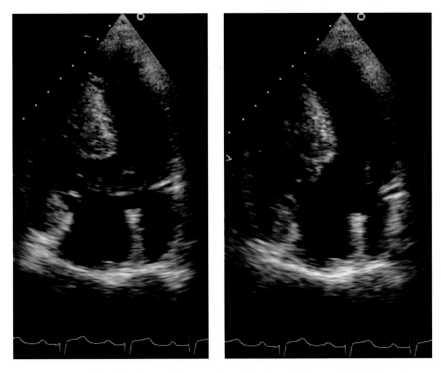

Figure 1.29. Apical four chamber view from a patient with atrioventricular septal defect. Note the ventricular and atrial components of the defect along with the common atrioventricular valve.

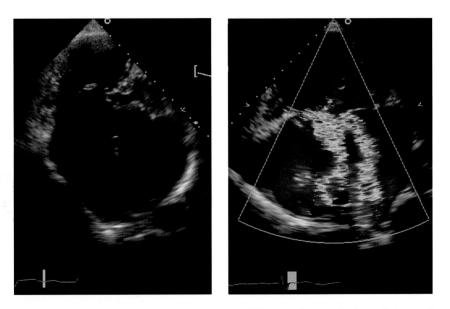

Figure 1.30. Apical four chamber view from a patient with Down syndrome and atrioventricular septal defect. Note significant atrioventricular valve regurgitation on color flow Doppler.

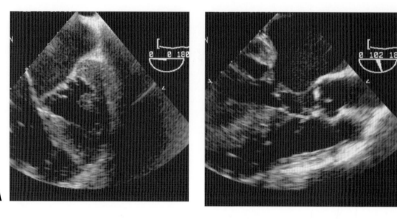

FIGURE 1.31. (A) Transesophageal echocardiographic four chamber view from a patient with repaired atrioventricular septal defect and (B) left ventricular outflow tract view demonstrating narrowed left ventricular outflow tract with significant obstruction and resulting marked left ventricle hypertrophy.

1.3.2. Follow Up

Echocardiography is the investigation of choice for assessing significant deterioration of atrioventricular valve regurgitation that may be the prime cause of symptoms in patients late after atrioventricular septal defect repair. Left ventricular outflow tract obstruction may also be present and/or progress after repair of the atrioventricular septal defects. Later, due to atrial dilatation, patients may develop atrial fibrillation which itself may contribute to ventricular dysfunction and pulmonary hypertension (see Figures 1.30 and 1.31).

2
Left Ventricular Inflow Obstruction

2.1. Cor Triatriatum

Cor triatriatum is a rare congenital cardiac anomaly in which a membranous structure divides the left atrium into two chambers. The distal chamber consists of pulmonary veins and the proximal chamber includes true left atrium and left atrial appendage. The communication between the pulmonary venous chamber and the rest of the atrium is usually restrictive; therefore, it commonly results in pulmonary venous congestion. The most common associated lesion with cor triatriatum is atrial septal defect. The atrial septal defect can either communicate with the pulmonary venous chamber or with the proximal chamber. A large secundum atrial septal defect or even two separate defects can communicate with the two chambers.

Adult patients with cor triatriatum who have no or mild symptoms may have very mild obstruction at rest. Obstruction may become obvious during stress and an increase in heart rate. When there is significant obstruction, patients usually present with secondary pulmonary hypertension. Associated mitral valve regurgitation can also be present. The mechanism for this is not well understood.

2.1.1. Echocardiographic Examination

Parasternal long-axis view shows a linear structure in the left atrium. Apical four chamber view demonstrates a membranous like structure in the left atrium that usually originates from the upper portion of the left lateral atrial wall. The insertion point on the septum is variable. The opening of the membrane can often be seen on two-dimensional images and color flow Doppler confirms its location and diameter. The degree of inflow narrowing can accurately be assessed by pulsed wave Doppler velocities. A low velocity of less than 1.2 m/s that demonstrates early and late diastolic components suggests no obstruction. In contrast, high early diastolic velocity that has lost its late component together with a dilated pulmonary venous chamber or large left-to-right shunt between pulmonary venous chamber and right atrium indicates significant obstruction.

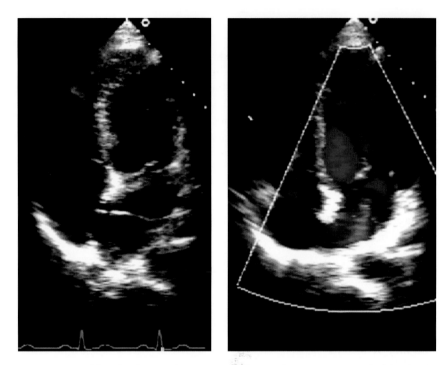

FIGURE 2.1. Apical four chamber view from a patient with a membranous structure in the left atrium.

Increased pulmonary artery pressure, which can be assessed from the peak tricuspid regurgitation velocity, is an indirect sign of significant obstruction. Patients with mild obstruction but dilated pulmonary venous chamber may develop significant obstruction during exercise. This can be clearly demonstrated by pharmacological stress echocardiography (see Figures 2.1 and 2.2).

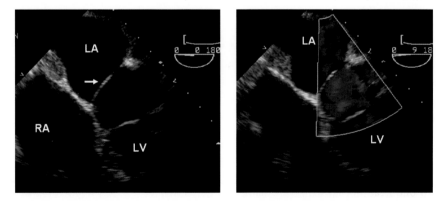

FIGURE 2.2. Transesophageal echocardiogram from a patient with cor triatriatum demonstrating an intra-atrial membrane that divides the left atrium into two chambers.

2.2. Supramitral Valve Membrane

This is a very rare condition in which an abnormally growing membrane between the left atrial appendage and the mitral valve leaflets is present. The level of the high velocity on color flow Doppler is usually shown above the mitral valve orifice level in the inflow tract. In patients with supramitral valve membrane, the mitral valve leaflets themselves are usually normal in anatomy and function. The parasternal long-axis view and apical four chamber view are ideal to demonstrate the lesion.

2.2.1. Management

Management of cor triatriatum and intra-atrial membrane is usually by surgical removal of the membrane as well as repair of the atrial septal defect.

2.3. Mitral Stenosis

Isolated mitral valve stenosis is one of the rarest forms of congenital heart disease. In adults, a variety of abnormal valve anatomy may be present and may contribute to the obstruction of blood flow from left atrium to left ventricle.

2.3.1. Double Orifice Mitral Valve

Double orifice mitral valve is a rare condition, often associated with atrioventricular septal defect. It is quite common for one of the two orifices to be either stenotic or regurgitant. If the diagnosis is suspected, the anatomical and physiological function of both orifices should be assessed. Double orifice mitral valve could remain a silent anomaly for years until valve incompetence becomes severe. At this stage valve repair may be considered in order to protect the left ventricle from functional deterioration.

Parasternal long and short-axis views of the mitral valve leaflets demonstrate the two orifices. In some cases, it may be difficult to demonstrate the two orifices in one echo plane (see Figure 2.3).

2.3.2. Parachute Mitral Valve

While normal mitral valve leaflets are supported by the anteromedial and posterolateral papillary muscles, parachute mitral valve is supported by either one papillary muscle, two fused papillary muscles, or three chordae attached to one head of papillary muscle. Although parachute mitral valve leaflets are anatomically abnormal, their function may be completely normal or only mildly stenosed.

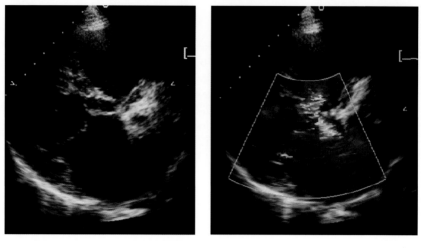

A   B

FIGURE 2.3. (A) Parasternal long-axis and short-axis views from a patient with double orifice mitral valve. (B) Note the presence of an incompetent orifice.

Parasternal long-axis view and apical four chamber view demonstrate the limitation of valve leaflets opening and subvalve narrowing. Short-axis view can demonstrate the chordal insertion into a single papillary muscle. Color Doppler shows the level of increase of flow velocity, not only at leaflets level, but also at subvalvar level (see Figures 2.4 and 2.5).

2.4. Mitral Valve Prolapse

Mitral valve prolapse is defined as the systolic billowing of one or both mitral valve leaflets into the left atrium. Congenital mitral valve prolapse is the most common cause of mitral regurgitation in adults. This lesion can be seen in isolation or in association with other anomalies, such as atrial septal defect or Marfan syndrome. Mitral valve prolapse and resulting regurgitation can be of variable degrees.

In patients with mild mitral valve prolapse, a midsystolic click is usually heard. It is caused by the backward mitral leaflet displacement in midsystole. This is often associated with late systolic mitral regurgitation, which is almost always mild in severity. Severity of mitral leaflet prolapse does not determine severity of mitral regurgitation. With severe regurgitation the murmur is usually short and peaks in midsystole (see Figure 2.6).

FIGURE 2.4. (A, B) Parasternal long- and short-axis views from a patient with a parachute left atrioventriclar valve. Note the chordal insertion into the posteromedial papillary muscle.

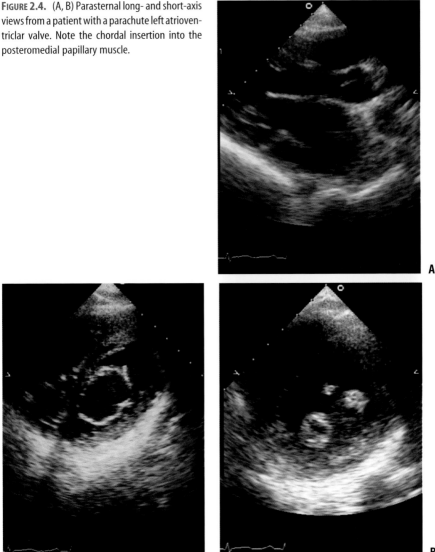

A

B

2.4.1. Assessment of Mitral Valve Regurgitation

2.4.1.1. Anatomical Diagnosis

This is easily achieved from transthoracic echocardiographic images and identification of the part of the leaflet that is prolapsing, in particular on the parasternal long-axis view. Good short-axis images may assist in determining the prolapsing scallop and its progressive dysfunction during follow up.

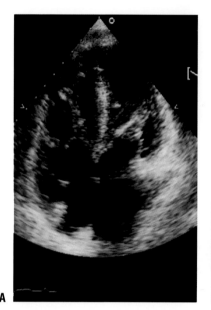
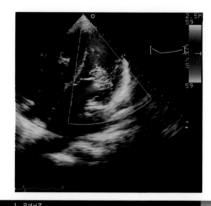
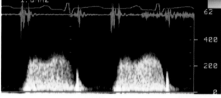

A   B

FIGURE 2.5. (A, B) Apical four chamber view of the same patient showing limited opening of the left atrioventricular valve. Color flow map showing turbulent flow starting at subvalve level and continuous wave Doppler demonstrating significant pressure gradient and important stenosis.

Transesophageal echocardiographic images may also help in delineating clearer images and accurate assessment of the exact prolapsing portion of the leaflet. Detailed assessment of the valve structure and function is crucial particularly when considering valve repair (see Figures 2.7 and 2.8).

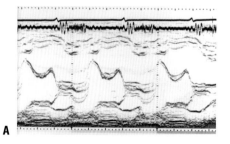
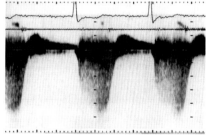

A   B

FIGURE 2.6. (A) M-mode echogram of the mitral valve prolapsing and (B) continuous wave Doppler showing late systolic mitral regurgitation, suggesting mild degree of regurgitation.

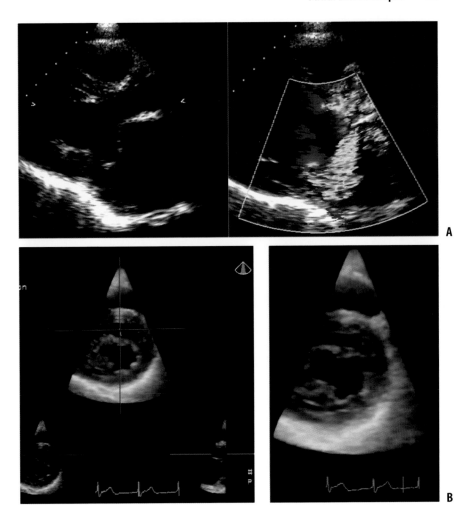

FIGURE 2.7. (A, B) Parasternal long-axis and three-dimensional short-axis view of the mitral valve from a patient with anterior mitral valve leaflet prolapse. Note the prolapsing mid-third of the anterior leaflet and resulting mitral regurgitation.

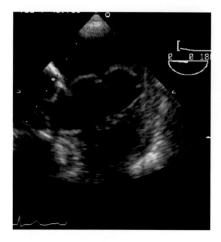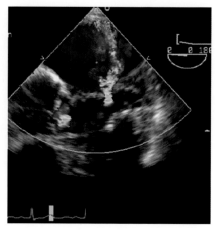

FIGURE 2.8. Transesophageal echocardiogram demonstrating posterior mitral valve leaflet prolapse causing mitral regurgitation.

2.4.1.2. Physiological Diagnosis

2.4.1.2.1. Color Flow Doppler

The degree of mitral regurgitation can be assessed by color flow Doppler based on:

1. **Jet Diameter.** A jet diameter at the leaflet tip level (vena contracta) broader than 5 mm suggests significant mitral regurgitation.
2. **Jet Area.** A mitral regurgitation jet area of more than 35% of the left atrial area is consistent with significant mitral regurgitation.
3. **Proximal Isovelocity Convergence Area (PISA).** This physiological principal estimates the degree of mitral regurgitation by measuring the diameter of the proximal velocity convergence at the leaflet tip level. This technique has its limitations, patients with displastic leaflets and those with distorted orifice may fail to demonstrate a clear spherical velocity convergence zone.

A common case for this is an eccentric mitral regurgitation jet, which is a common finding in patients with mitral valve prolapse. Therefore, color flow Doppler assessment of mitral regurgitation severity if taken in isolation may be misleading in these patients (see Figures 2.9 and 2.10).

2.4.1.2.2. Continuous Wave Doppler

Continuous wave Doppler is a very reliable technique for assessing severity of mitral regurgitation. Mild mitral regurgitation recordings display a decelerating

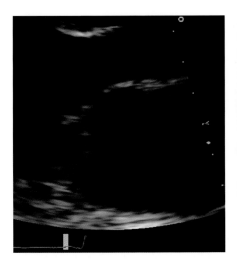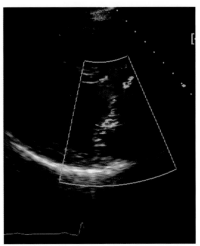

Figure 2.9. Parasternal long-axis view from a patient with posterior mitral valve leaflet prolapse that causes mild regurgitation with an anteriorly directed jet.

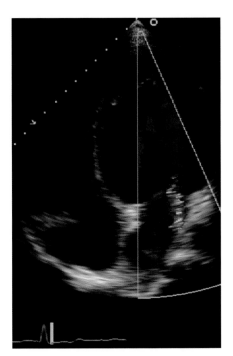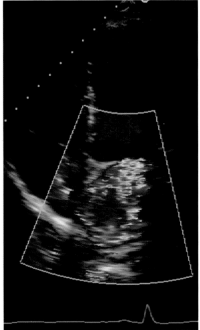

Figure 2.10. Apical four4 chamber view from two patients with mitral regurgitation on color Doppler, mild regurgitation (*left*) and severe regurgitation (*right*). Note the significant difference in jet diameter and area with respect to that of the left atrium.

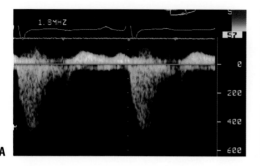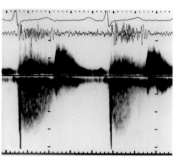

A   **B**

FIGURE 2.11. Continuous wave Doppler from a patient with (A) mild mitral regurgitation and another patient with (B) severe regurgitation. Note the difference in mitral regurgitation continuous wave Doppler signal, demonstrating early equalization of left atrial/left ventricular pressure, at end ejection in the patient with severe regurgitation.

pressure that extends well beyond end ejection (approximately 80 ms), whereas severe regurgitation demonstrates early equalization of left atrial and left ventricular pressures at end ejection (at the time of the second heart). Severe mitral regurgitation also results in suppression of systolic pulmonary venous flow component or even complete flow reversal. This sign should not be taken in isolation, particularly in patients with additional severe left ventricular systolic dysfunction. In them, mitral regurgitation peak pressure drop underestimates the driving left ventricular systolic pressure because of the raised left atrial pressure. Left atrial pressure in these circumstances can be estimated by subtracting the peak mitral regurgitation pressure drop from that of the systolic blood pressure (see Figure 2.11).

2.4.1.2.3. Left Ventricular Activity

Chronic overload of mitral regurgitation results in progressive increase in left ventricular dimensions, particularly in diastole. End systolic diameter always falls due to the large stroke volume, thus making conventional measurements of left ventricular systolic function from fractional shortening or ejection fraction erroneous. In patients who develop significant left ventricular disease and increase of end systolic volume, assessment of mitral regurgitation based only on left ventricular activity may underestimate severity of ventricular dysfuction (see Figure 2.12).

2.4.1.2.4. Management of Mitral Regurgitation

Mild mitral regurgitation is generally well tolerated by patients as long as left ventricular function is maintained. Management of severe mitral regurgitation

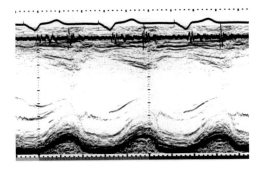

FIGURE 2.12. M-mode images of left ventricle cavity from a patient with severe mitral regurgitation. Note dilated left ventricle cavity size and active wall motion.

due to mitral valve prolapse is almost always by surgical leaflet repair with or without ring insertion, particularly in patients with posterior leaflet prolapse. Results of anterior leaflet repair is now very satisfactory in well-selected cases. In patients with chronic atrial fibrillation and severely dysmorphic mitral leaflets, valve replacement may be a better option. Simultaneous ablation of pulmonary veins has become a regular practice in these patients as an attempt to provide simultaneous treatment for the atrial arrhythmia.

2.4.1.2.5. Intraoperative Echocardiography

Intraoperative echocardiographic monitoring of mitral valve surgery has become a routine practice in most cardiac centres. Perioperative assessment of valve anatomy by transesophageal approach provides detailed anatomical imaging. Furthermore, any additional pathology that might have been missed preoperatively can be studied and assessed. A final careful examination of the valve function before closing the chest is crucial for excluding any residual lesion that should not be left uncorrected (see Figure 2.13).

2.4.1.2.6. Postoperative Follow Up

Transthoracic echocardiography provides an ideal means for postoperative follow up of patients after mitral valve surgery. The degree of residual or progressive valve regurgitation is assessed by different echocardiographic techniques, as mentioned above. Also, left ventricular dimensions, function, and activity are all assessed and quantified. In the absence of recurrent mitral regurgitation, significant increase in left ventricular end systolic volume or left atrial diameter represent increased ventricular stiffness and raised left atrial pressure as a possible cause for patient's breathlessness.

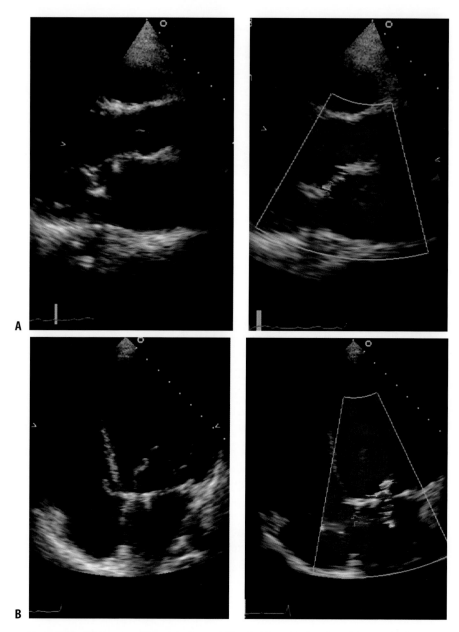

FIGURE 2.13. (A) Parasternal long-axis view and (B) apical four chamber view of the mitral valve from a patient after valve repair and insertion of a ring. Note the optimum repair and the valve competence postoperatively.

2.5. Partial Anomalous Pulmonary Venous Connections

Partial anomalous pulmonary venous connection is defined as the connection of one or more pulmonary veins to a site other than the morphological left atrium. It can occur as an isolated anomaly or in association with other intracardiac malformations. Here, we mainly discuss the anomalous connection in the setting of usual atrial arrangement. The connection can be described as totally or partially anomalous and unilateral or bilateral. When it is total, all four veins drain to the systemic circulation; when partial, some of the veins drain to the pulmonary circulation. The sites of anomalous connection are conventionally described as supracardiac, cardiac, and infracardiac. The most common type of supracardiac connection is for the pulmonary veins to join a confluence that drains through a common ascending vein to the brachiocephalic vein or directly to the right superior caval vein. The connection is described as cardiac when the veins insert directly into the right atrium or into the coronary sinus. In the infracardiac connection, the pulmonary veins usually converge to a horizontal confluence from which a vertical vein descends alongside the esophagus. This is also the type of connection most prone to stenosis and most challenging to repair.

The display of pulmonary venous anatomy may be complex, requiring interrogation from a number of transducer locations and planes. In the normal heart, the pulmonary veins may be seen from the subcostal, parasternal short-axis, suprasternal coronal, and apical four chamber views. In infants and small children, the pulmonary veins can be identified most readily from the subcostal location in the coronal view.

2.5.1. Subcostal Imaging

When the drainage site is below the diaphragm, the confluence tends to lie just below the diaphragm and is usually imaged with caudal angulation. The descending vein through the diaphragm usually drains through the esophageal hiatus. This route is anterior to and slightly rightward to the descending aorta, and posterior to and slightly leftward of the inferior vena cava. Thus, in this form of anomaly, three vascular structures drain through the diaphragm. When pulmonary venous drainage is intracardiac, either via the coronary sinus or directly into the right atrium, the draining confluence and the veins draining into it can be seen with more cranial angulation. With supracardiac pulmonary venous drainage, one must direct the subcostal transducer plane in the most cranial angulation. In addition to the confluence, it is important to identify all pulmonary veins draining into it. This can be aided by color flow Doppler and mapping of the region. When the drainage is to the superior caval system or directly to the right atrium, the plane must be directed in a most cranial direction from this transducer location.

2.5.2. Parasternal Imaging

The high parasternal short-axis view provides an alternative approach to image the pulmonary veins and the left and the right atria. The pulmonary veins lie between the pulmonary artery and left atrium and can be identified with cranial–caudal rocking of the transducer. Parasternal long-axis imaging is helpful for identifying the large coronary sinus. Color flow Doppler assists in identifying the exact location of the veins.

2.5.3. Suprasternal Imaging

In the suprasternal approach to imaging the anomalous pulmonary veins, their connection to a confluence and the site of drainage can also be achieved from the suprasternal notch. This may provide an excellent opportunity to image the vertical vein as it runs cranially or even to see its descent through the diaphragm.

2.6. Seimitar Syndrome

Seimitar syndrome is characterized by partial anomalous pulmonary venous drainage. The right-side pulmonary veins drain into the inferior vena cava and the left-side pulmonary veins usually drain into the left atrium. The right lung is almost always hypoplastic or completely absent, as well as the right bronchus. This syndrome is always associated with atrial septal defect and right cardiac chamber dilatation. Due to the hypoplastic right lung, the heart and the mediastinum tend to be shifted to the right.

2.6.1. Management

Management of Seimitar syndrome is by surgical repair of pulmonary venous drainage and the associated anomalies.

3
Left Ventricular Outflow Tract Lesions

3.1. Valvar Aortic Disease

Normal aortic valve is trileaflet. Congenital forms of valve disease are either unicuspid, bicuspid, or quadricuspid. Bicuspid valve is the most common congenital aortic valve disease, where the aortic valve is anatomically made of two leaflets or more but often functioning as bileaflet valve due to leaflet fusion. In this case, the overall valve function may be normal for years until late in life when calcification develops and the valve becomes stenotic or regurgitant. Although development of aortic stenosis or regurgitation of a bicuspid aortic valve is slow, fast deterioration can be triggered by endocarditis. This may destroy the valve and cause either significant stenosis or severe regurgitation. More than half of the patients with bicuspid aortic valve may present with aortic root dilatation partially due to intrinsic abnormality of aortic wall and partially due to poststenotic dilatation caused by eccentric jet.

3.1.1. Echocardiographic Examination

All echocardiographic views should be used to obtain detailed assessment of valve anatomy and function. Parasternal long-axis view is used to assess the valve mobility and cusp separation. The characteristic doming of the valve leaflets in systole is best seen from this view and the aortic root diameter can also be measured. Parasternal short-axis images are usually helpful in deciding on the number of aortic valve leaflets, particularly in the absence of significant calcification. Although true bicuspid aortic valve is easy to recognize from short-axis view, in some cases fusion of two of the three cusps would make the valve functionally bicuspid. These fused cusps display a raphe either between left and right coronary cusps or between left coronary and non-coronary cusp. The difference between functional bicuspid aortic valve and normal true trileaflet aortic valve is during systole when the valve opens. Functional bicuspid aortic valve opens like a fish mouth with certain degree of limitation of the leaflet excursion, while true trileaflet valve will move out freely and occupy a position near the wall of aortic root. In addition, the size of the cusps may vary from nearly equal to markedly different in area, so that closure line becomes eccentric. Due to the valve orifice position, which is often eccentric or slit-like, it is not usually possible to measure valve orifice area reliably by two-dimensional echocardiography.

The degree of valve stenosis can be assessed using continuous wave Doppler to achieve maximum transvalvar velocity from the apical five or three chamber views and to calculate peak instantaneous pressure difference (gradient) using the modified Bernoulli equation. The jet arising from a stenotic aortic valve may take many directions. To obtain the highest velocity one must interrogate the jet from a number of transducer positions to achieve optimal axial alignment. In some adults, right parasternal and suprasternal transducer position have to be used to acquire maximum transvalvar velocity. The peak instantaneous pressure difference calculated is frequently higher than peak-to-peak pressure difference recorded by catheter pull-back method.

Variable degrees of aortic regurgitation are often present with abnormal aortic valve. The degree of aortic regurgitation is best assessed by combined color and continuous wave Doppler, ventricular dimensions, and dynamic situation (see Figures 3.1 to 3.5).

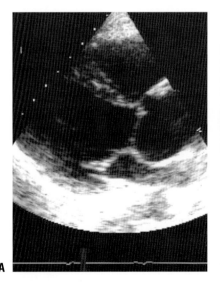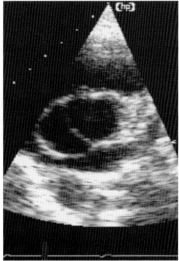

FIGURE 3.1. (A) Parasternal long-axis view from a patient with a bicuspid aortic valve showing thin leaflets with eccentric closure points. (B) Short-axis view demonstrating bicuspid aortic valve.

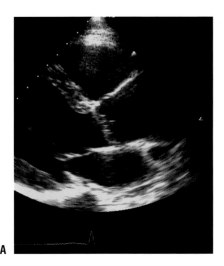
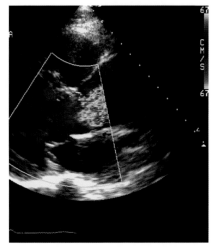

A   **B**

FIGURE 3.2. (A, B) Long- and short-axis views from a patient with a heavily calcified bicuspid aortic valve leaflets. Color Doppler shows turbulent flow across the valve.

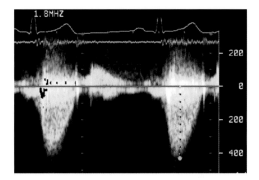

FIGURE 3.3. Continuous wave Doppler from the same patient showing significant aortic valve stenosis with a peak pressure drop of 70 mm Hg.

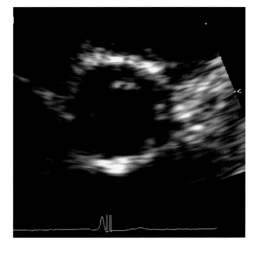

FIGURE 3.4. Parasternal short-axis view from a patient with a unicuspid aortic valve. Note the aortic orifice is in the middle of a single leaflet.

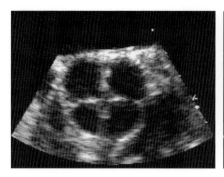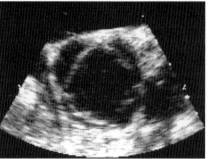

FIGURE 3.5. Parasternal short-axis view from a patient with a quadrileaflet aortic valve showing four leaflets and four commissures.

3.1.2. Management

3.1.2.1. Significant Valve Dysfunction, Stenosis, or Regurgitation

Mild and moderate aortic stenosis and regurgitation can be tolerated without significant symptoms. Severe valve stenosis or regurgitation need valve replacement surgery in order to avoid deterioration of ventricular function and to alleviate symptoms. Aortic valve substitute could be either mechanical or bioprosthesis. While the expected life of a mechanical valve is over 15 years, that of a bioprosthesis is in the order of 10 years. For young patients with isolated aortic valve disease, a homograft or autograft (patient's own pulmonary valve transferred to the aortic position, Ross Procedure) has proved ideal. In particular, the autograft has the advantage of growing with the patient. Symptomatic patients with only moderate valve dysfunction may benefit from stress echocardiography to assess the exact cause of symptoms and help plan appropriate management (see Figure 3.6 and 3.7). Recently, percutaneous aortic valve replacement has emerged as a new non-surgical treatment of aortic valve disease.

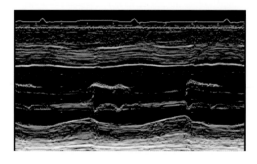

FIGURE 3.6. Left ventricular M-mode recording from a patient with significant bicuspid aortic valve stenosis showing left ventricular hypertrophy and dysfunction.

FIGURE 3.7. M-mode of left ventricular cavity from a patient who developed severe aortic regurgitation complicating bicuspid aortic valve disease. Note the increase in the diastolic 6.6 cm and systolic 4.6 cm dimensions and signs of deterioration of overall ventricular systolic function.

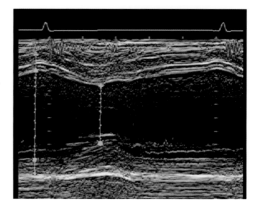

3.1.3. Complications

3.1.3.1. Endocarditis

The most serious complication in bicuspid aortic valve disease is endocarditis that triggers fast deterioration of valve function (see Figure 3.8).

3.1.3.2. Left Ventricular Disease

In addition to ventricular dilatation and deterioration of systolic function resulting from valve regurgitation, independent left ventricular disease can also develop with dilatation and dysfunction disproportionate to the severity of valve disease. This stage of ventricular disease is difficult to predict using conventional parameters (see Figure 3.9).

3.1.3.3. Aortic Root Dilatation

Dilatation of the aortic root is commonly seen and is known to be a progressive complication in bicuspid aortic valve disease and in some it may cause aortic

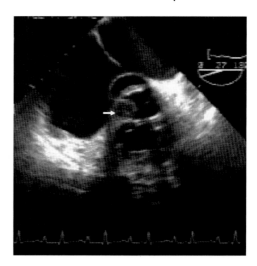

FIGURE 3.8. Transesophageal echocardiography from a patient with bicuspid aortic valve disease showing large vegetation on the valve cusps and abscess formation in the aortic root.

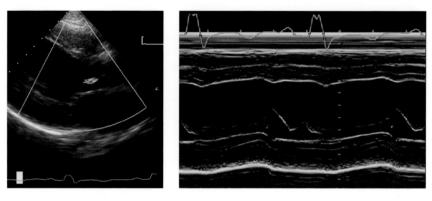

A   B

FIGURE 3.9. (A) Long-axis view of the left ventricle from a patient with a bicuspid aortic valve and aortic regurgitation. Note the disproportionate cavity dilatation and impairment of systolic function. (B) M-mode recording from the same patient.

dissection or even rapture. The generally accepted mechanism for the dilatation is eccentric jet lesion that causes dismorphic and fibrosed root. Recent data suggest that such patients who present with aortic root or ascending aorta dilatation have histological evidence for congenital aortic wall disease with early development of medial necrosis. Regular follow up of those patients with increased aortic root measurements is always recommended (see Figure 3.10).

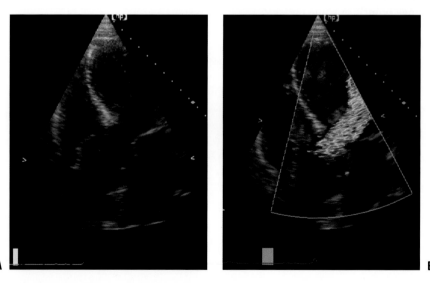

A   B

FIGURE 3.10. (A) Apical five chamber view from a patient with a bicuspid aortic valve showing dilated aortic root of 5 cm in diameter and (B) severe aortic regurgitation on color Doppler.

3.2. Subvalvar Aortic Stenosis

Subvalvar aortic stenosis may be caused by (1) fibromuscular ridge, (2) complete outflow tract ring that involves the anterior mitral valve leaflet, or (3) tunnel-like narrowing of the outflow tract. Diffused tunnel-type narrowing is often seen in association with a small aortic root.

In patients with hypertrophic obstructive cardiomyopathy, left ventricular outflow tract obstruction is caused by the combination of upper septal hypertrophy and systolic anterior motion of the mitral valve leaflets.

In adults with previous surgical repair of congenital heart anomalies, subaortic stenosis may also develop during the follow-up period. In patients with repaired atrioventricular septal defect, subaortic stenosis may develop due to abnormal accessory left atrioventricular valve apparatus tissue, or abnormal insertion of papillary muscles. In those with repaired double-outlet right ventricle and repaired Fallot, or transposition of great arteries after arterial switch, subaortic stenosis may develop from posterior deviation of the infundibular septum or angled surgical patch.

3.2.1. Echocardiographic Examination

Subaortic pathology is usually clearly seen from parasternal long-axis view. Occasionally, apical two or five chamber view and subcostal view may provide better diagnostic images. The fibromuscular ridge usually lies just beneath the aortic valve. In patients with complete ring, there may be membranous ridge seen on the anterior mitral valve leaflet just opposite the septum (so-called hinge point). In some patients, the ridge is so close to the aortic valve that the stenosis appears to be valvar in nature. Pulsed wave Doppler is helpful in differentiating the level of obstruction.

The turbulent flow produced from subvalvar region may cause aortic valve thickening and deformity, which may lead to valve incompetence. Early systolic closure of the aortic valve and the fine flutter, due to turbulent jet, on M-mode echocardiography are characteristic findings.

In addition to the unique use of two-dimensional echocardiographic images for determining the shape and position of the subaortic narrowing, color flow mapping and pulsed wave Doppler can be used to define the origin of acceleration. Continuous wave Doppler detects peak and mean blood velocities across the left ventricular outflow tract, hence the corresponding peak and mean pressure drop can be calculated by using the modified Bernoulli equation (see Figures 3.11 and 3.12).

3.2.2. Management

Severe subaortic stenosis with pressure difference exceeding 70 mm Hg requires surgical excision. This condition may recur again years after surgery.

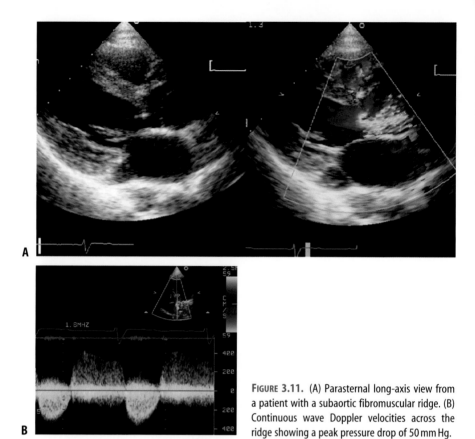

Figure 3.11. (A) Parasternal long-axis view from a patient with a subaortic fibromuscular ridge. (B) Continuous wave Doppler velocities across the ridge showing a peak pressure drop of 50 mm Hg.

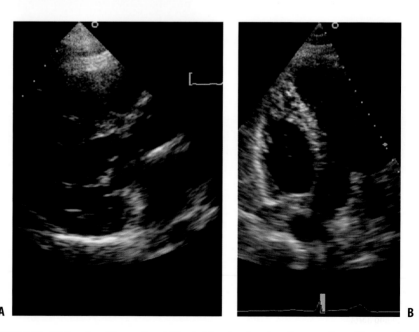

Figure 3.12. (A) Parasternal long-axis and (B) apical five chamber views from a patient with a complete outflow tract ring involving the anterior leaflet of the mitral valve.

Tunnel-like aortic root stenosis requires aortic root and valve replacement. Isolated valve replacement does not cure the condition.

3.3. Small Aortic Root

In this condition, there is no evidence for aortic leaflet disease but the aortic root itself and the proximal ascending aorta are small in size, less than 20 mm in diameter. The significant pressure difference across the aortic root requires root and valve replacement (see Figure 3.13).

3.3.1. Associated Abnormalities

3.3.1.1. Aortic Regurgitation

Aortic regurgitation is a common finding in patients with subaortic narrowing. It is due to the subaortic turbulant jet that hits the aortic valve, causing leaflet thickening and deformation and, hence, incomplete valve closure in diastole. There is growing evidence that patients with subaortic stenosis may have additional leaflet disease of varying degrees (see Figure 3.14).

Significant aortic regurgitation needs aortic valve replacement and excision of the subaortic shelf to protect the ventricle from functional deterioration.

3.3.1.2. Left Ventricular Hypertrophy

Left ventricular hypertrophy is a natural consequence to the outflow tract narrowing and increased pressure drop and cavity wall stress. The hypertrophy

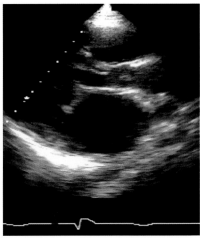
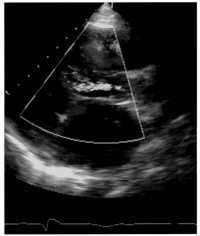

A   B

FIGURE 3.13. (A) Parasternal long-axis view from a patient with a small aortic root and ascending aorta and mild aortic regurgitation. (B) Note the tubular narrowing of the aortic root 20 mm just before the ascending aorta.

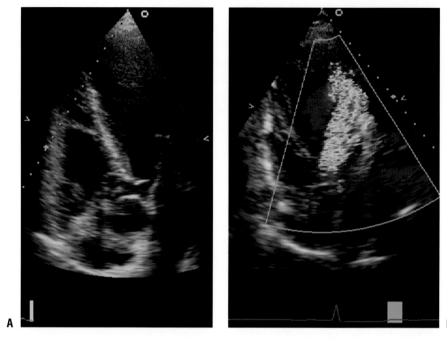

A   B

FIGURE 3.14. (A) Apical five chamber view from a patient with a subaortic ridge and (B) significant aortic regurgitation on color flow Doppler. Note the thicken aortic valve leaflets.

may regress after aortic valve replacement with improvement of overall ventricular function. The debate remains with regards to the best valve substitute that results in significant postoperative regression of left ventricular hypertrophy (see Figure 3.15).

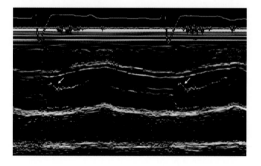

FIGURE 3.15. M-mode recording from a patient with subaortic stenosis showing premature aortic valve closure (arrow).

3.4. Supravalvar Aortic Stenosis

Supravalvar aortic stenosis is a rare condition where the aortic narrowing is at the level of the sinotubular junction. It may take the shape of an hourglass, narrowing at the proximal ascending aorta distal to the aortic sinuses. This anomaly is commonly seen in patients with Williams syndrome. It is complicated by calcification that tends to involve the aortic valve and aortic root. It may also involve the coronary artery orifices. The aortic narrowing can be part of a widespread arteriopathy affecting systemic and pulmonary arterial vessels.

3.4.1. Echocardiographic Examination

Parasternal long-axis view and suprasternal view with color flow mapping can identify the supra-aortic narrowing. From apical five chamber and suprasternal views using continuous wave Doppler, the peak flow velocity across the obstruction area can be obtained. Hence, the peak pressure difference can be calculated. With widespread arteriopathy, the aortic arch must be carefully examined in order to identify any branch vessel stenosis. Coexisting proximal pulmonary branch stenosis may also be identified from parasternal short-axis view. Distal branches of systemic and pulmonary arteries are better examined by magnetic resonance imaging (MRI) or contrast computed tomography (CT; see Figure 3.16).

Most patients with supra-aortic stenosis had often undergone complete repair early in life and they rarely develop recurrence. Some repaired cases may

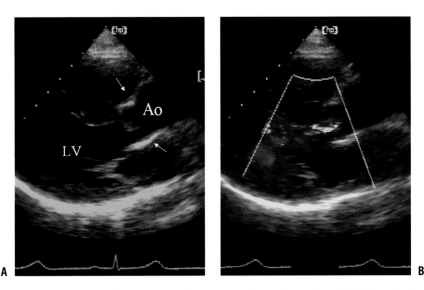

Figure 3.16. (A) Parasternal long-axis view showing supravalvar aortic stenosis and (B) mild aortic valve regurgitation on color flow Doppler from a patient with William syndrome.

develop left ventricular disease later in life. Associated aortic regurgitation may need long-term follow up.

3.5. Marfan Syndrome

Marfan syndrome is a connective tissue disease that involves multiple systems, such as cardiovascular, skeletal, and occular, to variable degrees. Cardiovascular involvement mainly manifests as progressive aortic root dilatation and aortic wall dissection. Mitral valve prolapse may also be seen in some cases.

3.5.1. Echocardiographic Examination

Echocardiography is the ideal investigation for examining cardiac involvement in Marfan syndrome and for the follow up of various lesions. Aortic diameters are usually measured at four levels: aortic annulus, sinus of Valsalva, sinotubular junction, and ascending aorta. Although beta blockers are usually prescribed to these patients for prophylactic support, progressive dilatation of the aortic root or ascending aorta to more than 55 mm irrespective of an evidence for dissection is an indication for a need for surgical repair. Elective aortic root surgery should be considered in patients who are at high risk of dissection irrespective of the aortic root diameter (e.g., family history of sudden death and females contemplating pregnancy). Recently, aortic exostent technique has

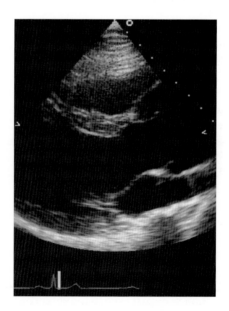

FIGURE 3.17. Parasternal long-axis view from a patient with Marfan syndrome showing dilated aortic root of 60 mm (this was accidentally found in a pregnant young woman).

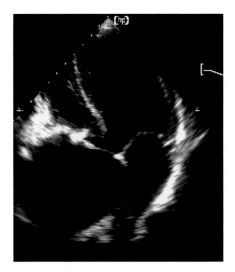 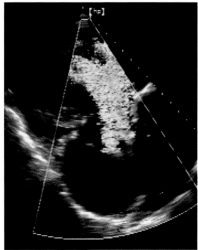

FIGURE 3.18. Apical five chamber view from the same patient showing significant aortic regurgitation on color flow Doppler.

been developed as an ideal procedure for them. Aortic root dilatation may result in aortic regurgitation. The degree of aortic valve regurgitation can be accurately assessed using color flow Doppler and continuous wave Doppler (see Figures 3.17 and 3.18).

Patients with Marfan syndrome may also present with aortic dissection although in some the aortic root itself may be normal in size. Transesophageal echocardiography is essential in assessing aortic dissection. The hallmark of a dissection is the intimal flap. In the longitudinal view, it may present as systolic expansion of the true lumen and compression of the false lumen. Color flow Doppler can help differentiate true and false lumens with low velocity flow in the latter; in addition, the entry and exit jets can often be seen. The false lumen may contain contrast echo and/or thrombus due to low velocity flow.

Transthoracic echocardiography is more useful in assessing complications, including aortic valve regurgitation due to aortic root dilatation or aortic rupture into the pericardium resulting in a pericardial effusion and temponade. In high-risk patients, a thorough assessment of the ascending and descending aorta using other imaging modality, such MRI or CT, is important, as the distinction between a proximal and distal dissection determines the need for surgical intervention (see Figure 3.19).

In a subgroup of patients with Marfan syndrome, coexisting left ventricle dilatation and dysfunction may exist even in the absence of aortic regurgitation. This needs to be thoroughly investigated and appropriately managed to avoid further deterioration of function.

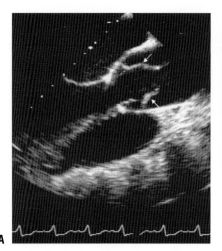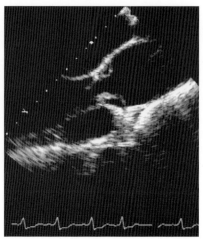

A   B

FIGURE 3.19. Parasternal long-axis view from a patient with Marfan syndrome showing a dissection flap (*arrows*) in the aortic root in (A) systole and (B) diastole.

3.6. Aneurysmal Aortic Root

This is a rare condition where the aortic root and/or sinuses become aneurysmal. The most serious complication of this condition is clot formation in the aneurysms with its potential consequences: coronary artery embolism, myocardial infarction, and aortic valve regurgitation (see Figure 3.20).

3.6.1. Sinus of Valsalva Aneurysms and Ruptured Sinus of Valsalva

The classical congenital sinus of Valsalva aneurysm is defined as the dilatation of one of the aortic sinuses between the aortic valve level and sinotubular junction. The right coronary sinus is the most common site for aneurysm formation. Non- and left coronary sinus dilatation are much less common. This lesion is often associated with ventricular septal defect, aortic regurgitation, and bicuspid aortic valve. Coronary artery anomalies may also be present. Progressive enlargement of the aneurysms may affect the adjacent structures and cause, right ventricular outflow tract obstruction.

Sinus of Valsalva aneurysms make the aortic wall weak and unstable; which in turn tends to progressively dilate and may finally rupture, particularly with increasing aortic pressure. The aneurysmal area is also a potential site of thrombus formation and infection.

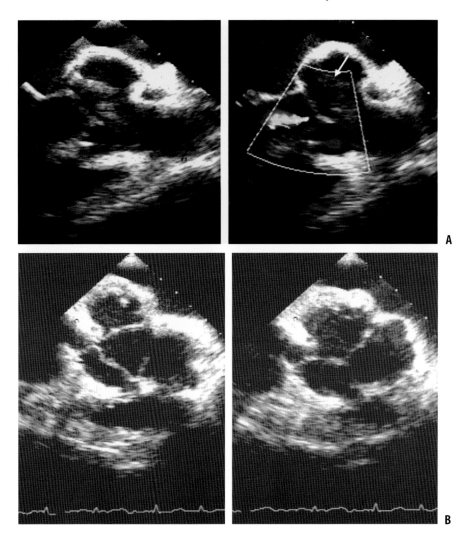

FIGURE 3.20. Transesophageal echocardiography showing (A) long- and (B) short-axis views from a patient with an aneurysmal aortic sinuses. Note the small clot (*arrow*) in the sinus cavity and the associated mild aortic regurgitation on color flow Doppler.

3.6.1.1. Echocardiographic Examination

Parasternal long- and short-axis views demonstrate the aneurysmal dilatation of the aortic sinuses. When there is an additional subaortic ventricular septal defect, the prolapsing aortic leaflet may partially close the defect and the corresponding sinus becomes distorted. This complex pathology often results in aortic regurgitation.

With ruptured sinus of Valsalva, the aneurysmal wall is discontinued, which can be seen on two-dimensional images. The ruptured tissue can have a wind-sock appearance and expand into right ventricular outflow tract. This may result in significant right ventricular outflow tract obstruction. The diagnostic feature is continuous flow from the aortic root into the connected chamber (usually the right ventricle) with relatively high velocity, The flow can also be confirmed on color flow Doppler and timed using color M-mode. The continuous pattern of the ruptured Sinus of Valsalva flow distinguishes it from ventricular septal defect flow, which is only systolic and aortic regurgitation which is only diastolic in timing (see Figures 3.21 and 3.22).

3.6.1.2. Management

Sinus of Valsalva aneurysm should be followed up regularly. The size of the aneurysm is measured on echocardiography and a coexisting lesion, such as ventricular septal defect, should be assessed. New onset of aortic regurgitation may mark the time for surgical repair. Ruptured sinus of Valsalva aneurysm with significant left-to-right shunt should be closed surgically or with a device.

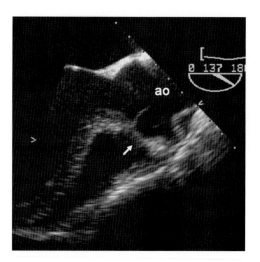

FIGURE 3.21. Transesophageal echocardiography of left ventricular outflow view showing the anerysmal dilatation of the right coronary sinus and prolapsing leaflet into the subaortic ventricular septal defect.

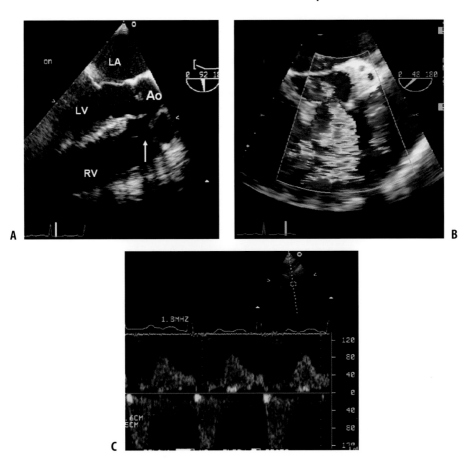

FIGURE 3.22. (A) Transesophageal echocardiography of the left ventricular outflow tract showing a ruptured sinus of valsalvar, (B) continuous flow on color Doppler, and (C) significant retrograde flow from descending aorta.

3.7. Postoperative Aortic Valve

It is generally accepted that patients with aortic valve replacement should be followed up annually by Doppler echocardiography. Early detection of valve dysfunction, stenosis, or regurgitation or ventricular disease should be documented and management optimized carefully. Valve substitutes determine the need for further surgical intervention.

3.7.1. Xenograft

Although the life expectancy of an aortic xenograft is 10 years, once the valve starts to degenerate its function deteriorates fast and an urgent need for revision surgery arises before the case becomes an emergency operation. The earliest signs of xenograft degeneration are leaflet redundancy or prolapse, progressive valve stenosis, or regurgitation. Transesophageal echocardiographic examination is usually essential in assessing the degree of valve dysfunction, as well as determining any evidence for proximal coronary artery obstruction, particularly in patients complaining of angina-like symptoms (see Figures 3.23 and 3.24).

3.7.2. Aortic Homograft

Aortic homografts are haemodynamically more stable than xenografts. They have approximately 10 years expected satisfactory performance. They avoid the need for anticoagulation.

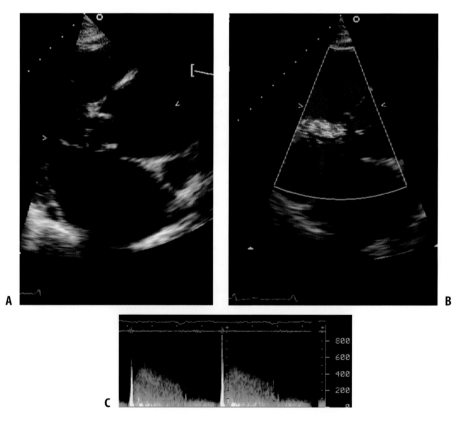

FIGURE 3.23. (A) Parasternal long-axis view from a patient with degenerating aortic xenograft, (B) color flow Doppler and (C) continuous wave Doppler showing significant aortic regurgitation.

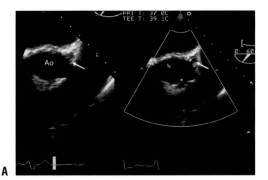
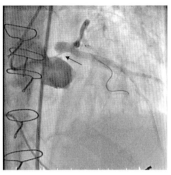

A   B

FIGURE 3.24. (A) Transesophageal echocardiogram demonstrating narrowed ostium of the left main coronary artery and turbulent flow on color flow Doppler (*arrow*). (B) Aortic root angiogram of same patient confirms echocardiographic finding.

3.7.3. Aortic Autograft (Ross Procedure)

Aortic autograft involves inserting the patient's own pulmonary valve in the aortic position and a homograft in the pulmonary position. This is a very successful operation, particularly for young patients, because it allows the valve to grow with the patient. Long-term follow up has been documented. When patients develop dysfunction, aortic regurgitation is the main presentation rather than stenosis. A velocity of 2.5 m/s across the pulmonary homograft months after the operation is a normal finding (see Figure 3.25).

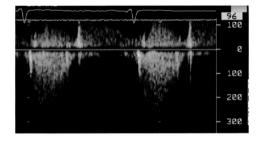

FIGURE 3.25. Continuous wave Doppler of the pulmonary homograft from a patient who underwent Ross procedure showing raised pulmonary homograft velocity less than 3 m/s.

3.7.4. Mechanical Valves

Mechanical valves are known for their durability. Recurrent infection around a mechanical valve ring suggests a need for replacement by a homograft. Patients with mechanical valves need to stay on anticoagulation indefinitely.

For further reading on mechanical valves, please refer to Springer's *Clinical Echocardiography* by Henein and colleagues and the Oxford *Textbook of Medicine*.

4
Disease of the Aorta

4.1. Patent Ductus Arteriosus

Patent ductus arteriosus is a blood vessel connecting the proximal left pulmonary artery to the descending aorta just distal to the left subclavian artery. During fetal life, the ductus arteriosus is a vital structure that bypasses the pulmonary circulation. A persistent shunt that remains patent well after birth is usually managed either surgically or interventionally by device (mostly coils) implantation early in life. Most adult cases with patent ductus arteriosus are small or silent without clinical hemodynamic significance. Moderate-sized ductus with significant left-to-right shunt causes left heart enlargement, and some degree of pulmonary hypertension are rarely seen. Large ducts in adults usually result in Eisenmenger physiology with eventual right-to-left shunt that may not be easy to diagnose using echocardiography. These patients have distal (lower body) cyanosis and toe clubbing.

4.1.1. Echocardiographic Examination

A parasternal sagittal ductus cut (in infraclavicular location in the second left intercostal space) demonstrates the ductus between the anteriorly located main pulmonary artery and posterior descending aorta. Ductus can also be visualized from the parasternal short-axis view. In this view, the ductus is imaged as a connection between the bifurcation of the pulmonary artery and descending aorta, attention is required not to mistake the left pulmonary artery for the ductus. Although short-axis view is a less reliable plane for demonstrating the ductus, color Doppler is of great help in demonstrating left-to-right shunt in patients with small ductus.

Left atrial and ventricular dilatation are the indirect signs of a significant left-to-right shunt. Continuous wave flow across the ductus reflects the pulmonary pressure. Tricuspid regurgitation velocity accurately reflects the pressure difference between the right ventricle and right atrium, from which the pulmonary artery pressure can be estimated (see Figure 4.1).

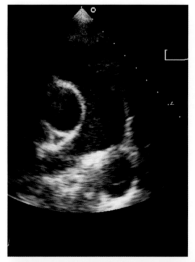
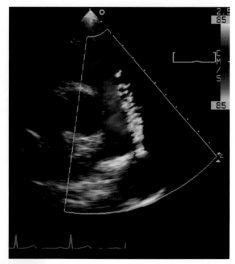

A

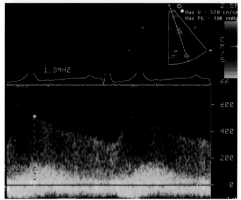

FIGURE 4.1. (A, B) Parasternal short-axis view showing a small duct on color flow Doppler. Note the characteristic (continuous) ductal flow on continuous wave Doppler.

B

Large ducts resulting in Eisenmenger syndrome will be discussed in a separate chapter.

4.2. Coarctation of Aorta

Aortic coarctation is defined as a narrowing or obstruction of the aortic arch. The region of the aortic arch frequently affected is that between the origin of the left subclavian artery and the insertion of the arterial duct, the region known as the isthmus. Two major variants of morphological coarctation, tubular hypoplasia and discrete coarctation, are recognized and the two may coexist.

Aortic coarctation can be best imaged from the high parasternal or suprasternal parasagittal plane. Discrete coarctation is characterized by a shelf of echo-dense tissue obstructing the aortic lumen from its posterior aspect. This shelf is usually located just distal to the origin of the left subclavian artery. In some patients, coarctation is associated with hypoplasia of the proximal aortic arch, as well as with the presence of additional stenosis in the region of transverse aorta and proximal descending aorta, or with a patent ductus arteriosus. Doppler is very helpful in assessing the severity of the coarctation. Direct interrogation of the site by continuous wave Doppler is characteristic. The high systolic velocity, which may continue throughout the cardiac cycle (diastolic tail) is characteristic of severe coarctation. Pulsed wave Doppler velocities of the descending aorta from the subcostal sagittal plane demonstrate reduced systolic flow, a characteristically low peak velocity, and prolonged acceleration and deceleration times. Studies have shown close relationship between systolic and diastolic velocities across the coarctation. Even in patients with pinpoint coarctation, the systolic velocity alone might underestimate the severity of the narrowing but diastolic velocity in the descending aorta represents a better marker for accurate assessment.

4.2.1. Management

While traditional treatment of aortic coarctation used to be surgical repair, percutaneous aortic coarctation stenting has become an attractive alternative with promising results (see Figures 4.2 and 4.3).

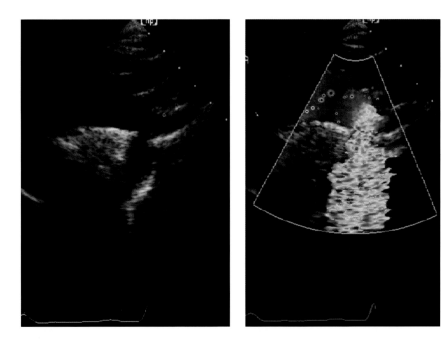

FIGURE 4.2. Two-dimensional suprasternal view of the aortic arch and proximal descending aorta from a patient with coarctation of the aorta demonstrating discrete narrowing.

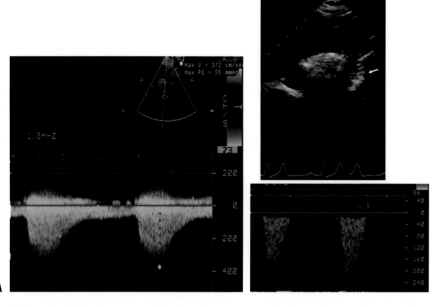

FIGURE 4.3. (A) Continuous wave Doppler velocities across the descending aorta from a patient with coarctation of the aorta demonstrating the characteristic flow pattern, high systolic velocity, and continuous flow during diastole with a velocity exceeding 2 m/s. (B) After stent insertion (*arrow*) to release the coarctation, there is a significant fall in both systolic and diastolic velocities.

4.3. Interruption of the Aortic Arch

This lesion is characterized by an absence of a segment of the aortic arch. Interruption of the aortic arch may occur at one of three different levels: beyond the left subclavian artery (type A), between the left common carotid and left subclavian arteries (type B, most commom), or between the innominate and the left common carotid artery (type C). Echocardiographic features of this lesion include hypoplasia of the ascending aorta and of the proximal arch, an area of discontinuity between the proximal arch, and a descending aorta. The interruption of the aortic arch is best imaged from the suprasternal view; however, high parasternal views are also a good approach in infants and children. Determination of the flow direction and pattern in the arch vessel by color Doppler and pulsed wave Doppler is important for establishing the diagnosis. Interruption of the aortic arch is almost always associated with other congenital cardiovascular lesions, including patent ductus arteriosus, ventricular septal defects, truncus arteriosus, and aortopulmonary window.

4.4. Common Arterial Trunk

The common arterial trunk is characterized by a single arterial vessel arising from the base of the heart, through a common arterial valve, which gives origin directly to the systemic, pulmonary, and coronary arteries. The lesion is classified into four types based on the origins of the pulmonary arteries. In type I, the common pulmonary artery arises from the trunk and divides into left and right pulmonary arteries. In type II, both right and left pulmonary arteries arise close together from the left-posterior aspect of the trunk. In type III, the pulmonary arteries arise separately from the right and left lateral aspects of the trunk. Type IV has been classified as an entity where no pulmonary vessels arise from the ascending aorta, but pulmonary vessels arise from the descending aorta, although this type is not considered by many to be a form of common arterial trunk. In most cases, there are concordant atrioventricular connections and the cardiac septum is well formed apart from a large outlet ventricular septal defect. Rarely, it is associated with an atrioventricular septal defect.

From the parasternal long-axis view, there is a large single vessel and variable degrees of overriding of the ventricular septum. This finding is similar to other forms of conotruncal defects, such as tetralogy of Fallot and double outlet right ventricle. On echocardiographic examination, the truncal valve is very often deformed and thickened. The parasternal short-axis images provide the best view for defining the valve cusps. The truncal valve is frequently tricuspid but has been reported to have from two to six cusps. The presence of restricted valvar opening reflects the degree of truncal valve stenosis. The significance of truncal valve stenosis and regurgitation can be assessed by color and continuous wave Doppler similar to that used to assess the aortic valve. Ventricular septal defect in this condition is usually in an outlet position and the atrioventricular valves are of normal offsetting. The defect can be imaged from a variety of parasternal, apical, and subcostal regions (see Figures 4.4 and 4.5).

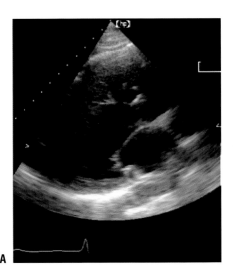 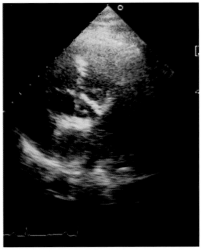

A   B

FIGURE 4.4. (A) Parasternal long-axis view and (B) short-axis view from a patient with common arterial trunk demonstrating the truncal override and the single artery. Note the four leaflet truncal valve in the short-axis images in this case.

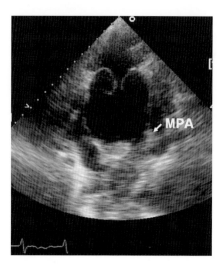

FIGURE 4.5. Parasternal short-axis view from a patient with truncus arteriosus showing the classical diagnostic features of type I truncus.

5
Tricuspid Valve Abnormalities

5.1. Ebstein Anomaly

Ebstein malformation is the most common form of congenital tricuspid valve disease. It is defined as apical displacement of parts of the hinge point of the tricuspid valve leaflets, within the right ventricular cavity and away from the atrioventricular junction. It is almost always accompanied by dysplasia of the leaflets. Leftward and inferior displacement of the proximal attachment is the most common form of Ebstein anomaly that may involve the septal and posteroinferior (mural) leaflets, whereas the anterosuperior leaflet is usually normally attached, but enlarged with a sail-like appearance.

The displacement of the septal leaflet of the tricuspid valve is best displayed in the apical four chamber view. Normally, the septal tricuspid leaflet inserts only slightly (10 mm) toward the apex in comparison with the anterior (aortic) mitral valve leaflet. The degree of displacement can be determined by measuring the distance between mitral and tricuspid septal insertion offset and the apex or the direct distance between the two points of insertion. The mobility of the tricuspid valve leaflets is also reduced in Ebstein anomaly. Displacement of the posteroinferior leaflet can be demonstrated in the subcostal coronal and sagittal views. Parasternal long-axis views with medial angulation to image the right ventricle may also display the tethering of the posteroinferior leaflet to its underlying myocardium. The anterosuperior leaflet is usually well demonstrated in several planes. The proximal segment of the anterosuperior leaflet is commonly attached to the atrioventricular groove, which can clearly be demonstrated in the apical four chamber view. As a result of the tricuspid valve leaflet displacement, the atrialized portion of the right ventricle becomes large, adding to the dilatation of the right atrium caused by tricuspid regurgitation. The most frequent additional anomaly seen in Ebstein malformation is atrial septal defect.

Ebstein anomaly is almost always associated with significant tricuspid valve regurgitation. This can easily be confirmed by color Doppler, as it demonstrates a large regurgitation jet originating down in the right ventricular cavity near the apex and fills the atrialized right ventricle and the true right atrium. Color flow aliasing should not be taken as a diagnostic feature because with severe regurgitation velocities might be too low to alias. Color Doppler flow may also

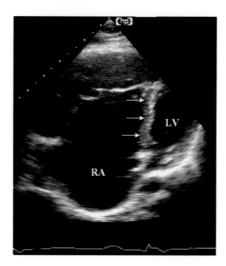

FIGURE 5.1. Apical four chamber view from a patient with Ebstein anomaly demonstrating a 4-cm apical displacement of the septal tricuspid valve leaflet below the valve annulus level. Note the sail-like appearance of the anterosuperior leaflet, which is characteristic of this anomaly.

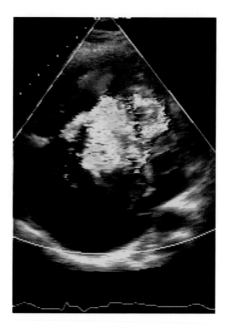

FIGURE 5.2. Color flow Doppler from the same patient demonstrating large regurgitant jet that originates near the right ventricular apex and fills the whole of the atrialized right ventricle and the true right atrium.

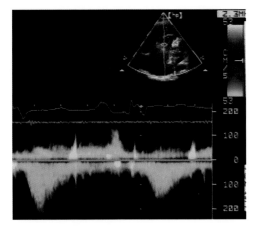

FIGURE 5.3. Continuous wave Doppler recording of tricuspid regurgitation from the same patient demonstrating all signs of severity: low retrograde pressure drop and pressure equalization between the right ventricle and right atrium at end ejection.

demonstrate more than one valve orifice towards the ventricular apex. Continuous wave Doppler detects tricuspid regurgitation that is almost always severe. Signs of severity are low retrograde velocity and pressure drop across the tricuspid valve (due to raised right atrial pressure) that underestimates systolic right ventricular pressure, equalization of right ventricular and right atrial pressure drop at end ejection, and laminar flow pattern (on pulsed wave Doppler) of the tricuspid regurgitation flow. Pulsed wave Doppler recordings of superior and inferior vena caval flow demonstrates systolic flow reversal and dominant early diastolic filling of the right atrium (see Figures 5.1, 5.2, and 5.3).

5.2. Tricuspid Valve Prolapse

Congenital tricuspid valve prolapse that causes tricuspid regurgitation is very rare, but still seen. Tricuspid valve prolapse can also result from myocardial infarction or blunt chest trauma, causing rupture of the papillary muscle or chordae. Sometimes, the leaflets themselves are dysplastic—one of the leaflets is shortened and tethered and prevents prompt valve closure during systole. Three-dimensional echocardiographic images are very helpful in identifying the prolapsing leaflet and estimating severity of tricuspid regurgitation (see Figures 5.4 and 5.5).

5.3. Tricuspid Valve Stenosis

Congenital tricuspid stenosis can be due to underdeveloped annulus, shortened chordae, valve fused commissures, hypoplastic and calcified leaflets, parachute deformity, and a supravalvar membrane (see Figures 5.6, 5.7, and 5.8).

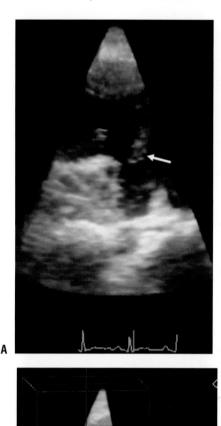

A

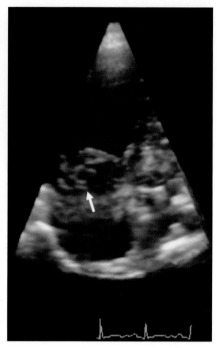

B

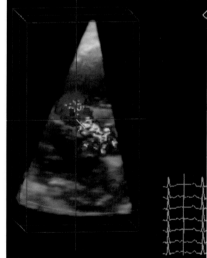

C

FIGURE 5.4. (A) Three-dimensional echocardiographic images of right ventricular inflow; (B) four chamber view of a prolapsing tricuspid valve, and (C) three-dimensional color Doppler showing tricuspid regurgitation.

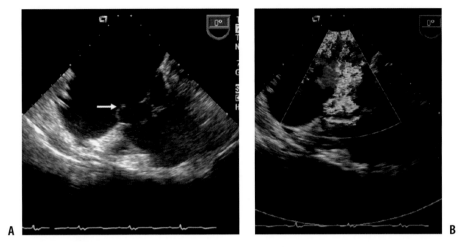

Figure 5.5. (A) Transesophageal echocardiogram showing tricuspid valve prolapse (*arrow*) and (B) tricuspid regurgitation on color Doppler.

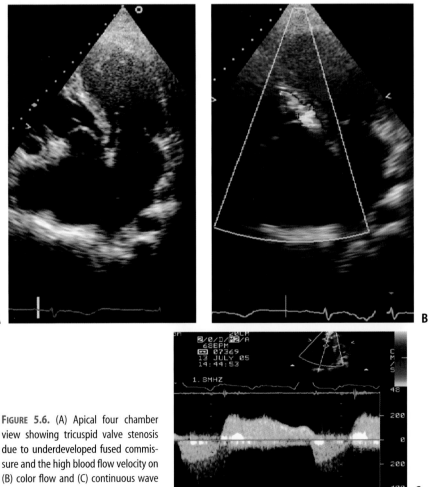

Figure 5.6. (A) Apical four chamber view showing tricuspid valve stenosis due to underdeveloped fused commissure and the high blood flow velocity on (B) color flow and (C) continuous wave Doppler recordings.

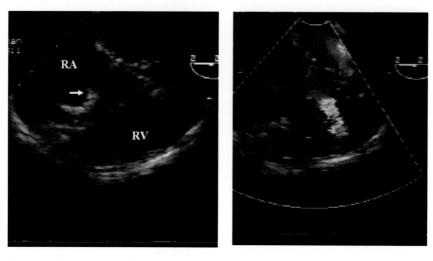

FIGURE 5.7. Transesophageal echocardiongram showing tricuspid valve stenosis due to calcified valve leaflet. Tricuspid valve stenosis is also seen in patients post surgical valve annuloplasty or valve replacement.

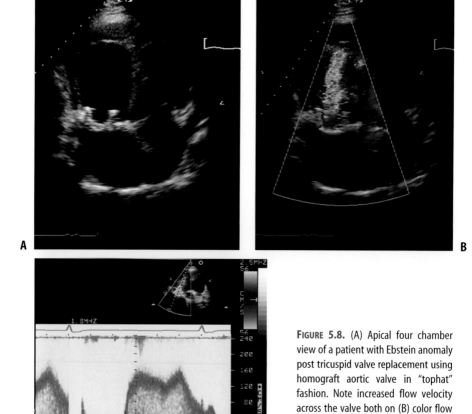

FIGURE 5.8. (A) Apical four chamber view of a patient with Ebstein anomaly post tricuspid valve replacement using homograft aortic valve in "tophat" fashion. Note increased flow velocity across the valve both on (B) color flow Doppler and (C) pulsed wave Doppler, suggesting relative valve stenosis.

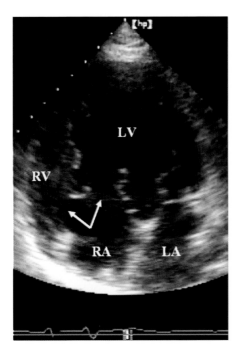 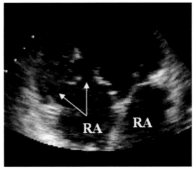

FIGURE 5.9. Apical four chamber view of a patient with double inlet left ventricle with inlet ventricular septal defect and hypoplastic right ventricle. Note the right atrioventricular valve has two orifices.

5.4. Double Orifice Tricuspid Valve

Double orifice tricuspid valve is a very rare condition, mostly seen in patients with atrioventricular septal defects, and occasionally in more complex congenital heart defects (see Figure 5.9).

6
Right Ventricular Outflow Tract Lesions

6.1. Pulmonary Valve Stenosis and Regurgitation

Valvar pulmonary stenosis can present as isolated congenital anomaly or as part of other complex congenital heart abnormalities, such as tetralogy of Fallot, transposition of great arteries, or syndromes such as Noonan syndrome.

Pulmonary valve stenosis may result from commissural fusion, valve or leaflets dysplasia, or bicuspid valve abnormality. The echocardiographic diagnosis of pulmonary valve stenosis is based on several features that can be defined using a variety of views and ultrasound modalities. In adults, parasternal long-axis view with leftward tilt of the transducer, parasternal short-axis view, and, in some cases, apical five chamber view with further anterior angulation are the useful views to demonstrate the pulmonary valve and its function. The valve leaflets are usually thickened and doming. When the valve is calcified, the leaflets become densely reflective with limited excursion. Color flow Doppler demonstrates narrowed turbulent flow jet across the pulmonary valve. Continuous wave Doppler can detect increased flow velocity, from which peak pressure drop across the valve can be calculated using the modified Bernoulli equation (pressure drop = $4V^2$). Variable degrees of poststenotic dilatation of the main pulmonary artery are often seen in adult patients. Right ventricular hypertrophy secondary to pulmonary stenosis is another feature. Sometimes the right ventricular hypertrophy from longstanding severe pulmonary valve stenosis results in significant right ventricular infundibular obstruction by the hypertrophied muscle. In such cases, continuous wave Doppler demonstrates double density signal or late peak flow velocity from the infundibular stenosis. Despite the significant hypertrophy, right ventricular systolic function is often maintained. As is the case with left ventricular hypertrophy, longstanding hypertrophy of the right ventricle, increases wall stress, leading to subendocardial ischemia and eventually results in stiff cavity and raised end diastolic pressure. This is reflected on the pattern of ventricular filling that becomes restrictive, consistent with raised right atrial pressure. The raised right atrial pressure and right atrial stretch, in turn, predisposes to arrhythmia. Also, the continuous rise in right atrial pressure will be reflected on the systemic pressure and hence may cause fluid retention. The echocardiophic features of restrictive right ventricular physiology are large "*a*" wave on transpulmonary Doppler presented throughout respiration, large mechanical "*a*" wave on right ventricle long-axis excursion as demonstrated by M-mode echocardiography, and small Doppler "*a*" wave on transtricuspid flow. Large "*a*" wave on Doppler recording of the SVC and increased retrograde flow velocity during atrial systole on SVC or IVC (superior vena cava or inferior vena cava) Doppler are also additional diagnostic features of right ventricular restriction.

Pulmonary valve regurgitation is often seen in patients who had previous pulmonary valvotomy (surgical or ballooning). With severe pulmonary regurgitation, patients often develop progressive right ventricular dilatation from the volume overload and tricuspid annulus dilatation and tricuspid valve regurgitation (quantification of pulmonary regurgitation is discussed in detail in Chapter 7; see Figures 6.1, 6.2, and 6.3).

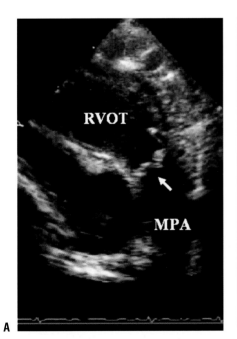
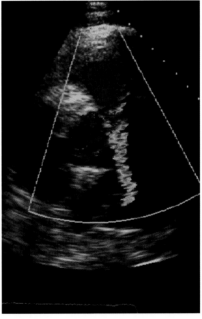

A   **B**

FIGURE 6.1. (A) Short-axis views from a patient with congenital pulmonary valve disease showing thickened and doming leaflets and (B) turbulent flow across the valve, suggesting valve stenosis.

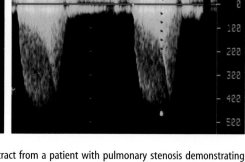

FIGURE 6.2. (A) Right ventricular outflow tract from a patient with pulmonary stenosis demonstrating additional subvalvar narrowing caused by muscle hypertrophy. (B) Continuous wave Doppler from the same patient demonstrating double velocity pattern consistent with two levels of narrowing in right ventricular outflow tract.

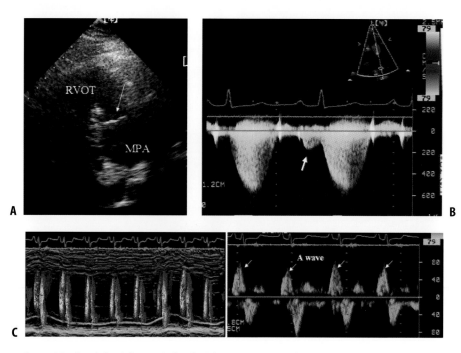

FIGURE 6.3. Restrictive right ventricular physiology in a patient with Noonan syndrome and pulmonary stenosis post pulmonary valvotomy. Note the thickened pulmonary valve leaflets on (A) a wave (*arrow*) on the pulmonary flow (B) and late diastolic retrograde flow in IVC (C).

6.2. Double Chamber Right Ventricle

6.2.1. Definition

Double chamber right ventricle is characterized by a prominent muscular band in the right ventricle that divides the cavity into two chambers. This may result in the development of intracavitary pressure gradient. The severity of obstruction can vary considerably and may be underestimated when the Doppler signal is not parallel to the accelerated flow jet.

Parasternal short-axis view can demonstrate the right ventricular body and the hypertrophied muscle bundles. The flow jets both on color and continuous wave Doppler can easily be misinterpreted with the flow across a ventricular septal defect. Color flow imaging or pulsed wave Doppler interrogation within the right ventricular outflow tract may help in defining the condition. Apical five chamber view with further anterior angulation may demonstrate clearly the

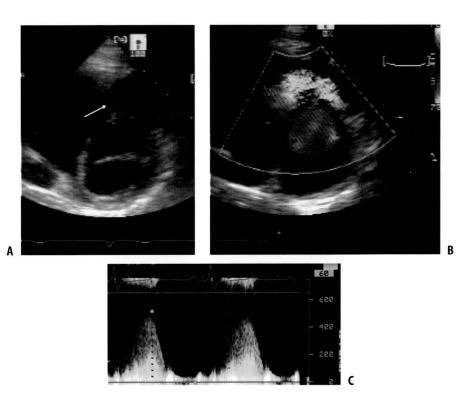

A   B

                                                                C

FIGURE 6.4. (A) Parasternal short-axis view demonstrating a muscle band (*arrow*) that divides the right ventricle into two chambers, and (B) respective color, and (C) continuous wave Doppler velocities, suggesting significant obstruction.

right ventricular outflow tract region and may assist accurate recording of the peak velocity across the obstruction area. In children, subcostal coronal and sagittal views can display the abnormal muscle bundle.

A very high incidence of associated perimembranous ventricular septal defect has been reported. With double chamber right ventricle, the ventricular septal defect may open into the high or low pressure chamber of the right ventricle. When it opens into the high pressure chamber, the shunt may not be seen. Double chamber right ventricle may be differentiated from infundibular obstruction by the presence of trabeculae in the distal chamber (see Figures 6.4 and 6.5).

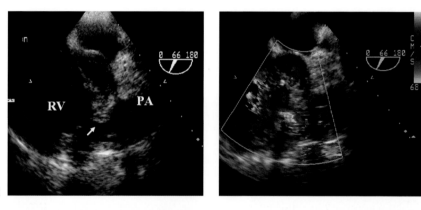

FIGURE 6.5. Transesophageal echocardiogram of right ventricular inflow and outflow view showing the relationship between the muscle band (*arrow*), the exact site of narrowing and the pulmonary valve. Note the presence of trabeculae in the distal chamber.

7
Other Congenital Heart Diseases with Major Right Ventricular Involvement

7.1. Tetralogy of Fallot

Tetralogy of Fallot is the most common form of cyanotic heart anomalies, accounting for approximately 10% of all congenital heart diseases. In anatomic terms, this malformation consists of four components: subpulmonary infundibular stenosis, ventricular septal defect, overriding of the aorta, and right ventricular hypertrophy.

The hallmark of tetralogy of Fallot is an anterocephalic deviation of the outlet septum, causing subpulmonary obstruction in the right ventricular outflow tract. As a result of this malalignment, a ventricular septal defect exists in the subaortic region. Rightward deviation of the aortic orifice, with overriding of the valvar leaflets in relation to the crest of the ventricular septum is also part of this anatomy. Right ventricular hypertrophy is secondary to right ventricular hypertension.

Tetralogy of Fallot represents a wide morphological spectrum. At one end, it can be difficult to distinguish hearts with tetralogy of Fallot from those with ventricular septal defect and aortic overriding with mild pulmonary sternosis. At the other extreme, the pulmonary obstruction is so severe as to represent the most common variant of pulmonary atresia in the presence of a ventricular septal defect.

7.1.1. Natural History and Surgical Management

Twenty-five percent of patients with tetralogy of Fallot die in the first year of life if not surgically treated. Forty percent die before 3 years of age, 70% die before 10 years of age, and 95% die before 40 years of age. However, when the right ventricular outflow tract obstruction is mild, patients often have minimal cyanosis (so-called *pink tetralogy* or *acyanotic Fallot*) and may occasionally present in adulthood. Morbidity in adult survivors with unoperated tetralogy of Fallott is high and relates to progressive cyanosis, exercise intolerance, arrhythmia, tendency to thrombosis, and cerebral abscess. In those few naturally surviving into the fourth and fifth decades of life, death usually occurs due to congestive heart failure, secondary to longstanding right ventricular hypertension, or suddenly, presumably due to arrhythmia. Surgical repair of tetralogy of Fallot has improved long-term survival and life expectancy.

7.1.2. Echocardiographic Assessment

7.1.2.1. Unoperated Tetralogy of Fallot

Most adults will have had surgery, either palliative or, more commonly, reparative by the time they present in the adult cardiology clinic. Adults rarely present without previous operations.

7.1.2.1.1. Ventricular Septal Defect

The ventricular septal defect in tetralogy of Fallot is usually single and almost always large and nonrestrictive, except in very rare cases where its right ventricular margin is shielded by accessory tricuspid valve tissue or where marked septal hypertrophy narrows the defect. In about 80% of cases, the defect is perimembranous; the remainder have a muscular posteroinferior rim. Much less commonly, the defect can be doubly committed juxta-arterial, with its cephalic border formed by the aortic and pulmonary valves. The parasternal long-axis and short-axis views demonstrate the size and location of the ventricular septal defect (see Figure 7.1).

7.1.2.1.2. Pulmonary Stenosis

There is a degree of right ventricular infundibular stenosis in almost all cases of tetralogy of Fallot, which commonly coexists with obstructions at other sites. The anterocephalic deviation of the outlet septum and the hypertrophied septoparietal trabeculations constitute the major anatomic basis for the right

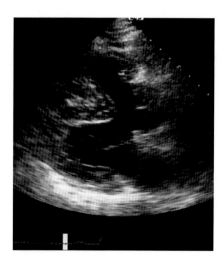

FIGURE 7.1. Parasternal long-axis view from a patient with tetralogy of Fallot demonstrating the relationship between the ventricular septal defect and the aortic root and valve. Note the significant right ventricular hypertrophy in this adult patient.

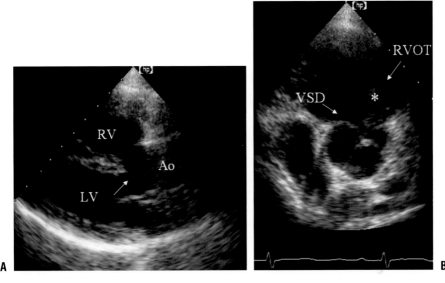

FIGURE 7.2. Parasternal long-axis (A) and short-axis (B) views from a patient with tetralogy of Fallot demonstrating the large subaortic ventricular septal defect, the overriding aorta, and the narrowed right ventricular outflow tract related to the deviation of the outlet septum (*).

ventricular outflow tract obstruction. The second level of subpulmonary obstruction is the hypertrophied moderator band and apical trabeculation, which produce more proximal stenosis and gives the arrangement of two-chambered right ventricle. The pulmonary valve itself is abnormal in most cases of tetralogy of Fallot. Acquired atresia of the infundibulum or the valve may also occur. Pulmonary artery stenosis may occur at branch points from the bifurcation onwards. Hypoplasia of the pulmonary arteries has been reported as frequently as in 50% of patients. Non-confluent pulmonary artery to the pulmonary trunk is not infrequent. The nonconnected pulmonary artery is almost always present, usually being connected by the arterial duct to some part of the aortic arch. Rarely, the pulmonary artery may arise directly from the ascending aorta, but it is more often the right pulmonary artery which is anomalously connected. In adults, the parasternal long-axis view with lateral angulation is valuable for imaging the right ventricular outflow, the pulmonary valve area, the main pulmonary artery, and the bifurcation (see Figure 7.2). This view is useful for studying Doppler velocities across the right ventricular outflow tract. Parasternal short-axis view can also display the area of the infundibular septum and its deviation to the right ventricular outflow tract. With slight angulation or more cranial or caudal transducer placement, the main pulmonary artery and its branches can be clearly displayed and the actual diameter of pulmonary arteries can be measured. It is important to examine the coronary

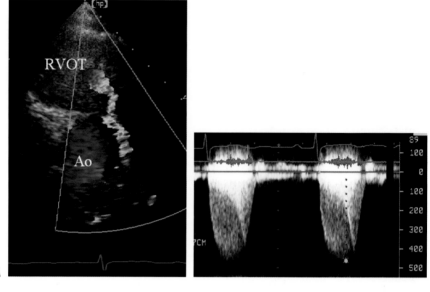

A   B

FIGURE 7.3. (A) Parasternal short-axis view from a patient with tetralogy of Fallot demonstrating the narrowed infundibulum as well as a small main pulmonary artery and branches. (B) Double shadowed continuous wave Doppler trace recorded from right ventricular outlet tract is characteristic of infundibular and valvar pulmonary stenosis.

arteries and their relationship to the right ventricular outflow tract in the short-axis view, although this may be difficult to achieve in adults (see Figure 7.3).

7.1.2.1.3. Aortic Overriding

The classical parasternal long-axis view is the best to image the aortic override of the ventricular septum. The degree of aortic override can vary from 5% to 95% of the valve being connected to the right ventricle. Tetralogy of Fallot, therefore, may coexist with double outlet right ventricle, when more than half (50%) of the aorta is connected to the right ventricle.

7.1.2.1.4. Associated Lesions

Patent foramen ovale, atrial septal defect, a second muscular ventricular septal defect, or an atrioventricular septal defect, usually in the setting of Down syndrome, and coarctation of aorta may coexist with tetralogy of Fallot. A right aortic arch is common and sometimes associated with anomalous origin of the subclavian artery. Coronary arterial abnormalities, such as a left anterior descending artery originating from the right coronary artery, crossing the right ventricular outflow tract, may occur in about 3% of patients and may be of surgical importance. This situation sometimes necessitates the use of a right ventricular-to-pulmonary artery conduit.

7.1.2.2. Patients with Palliative Procedures

There are occasional patients who may reach adulthood with a palliative procedure only. The types of different palliative procedures that augment pulmonary blood flow in tetralogy of Fallot are:

- **Blalock–Taussig shunt (Classical).** Subclavian artery to pulmonary artery anastomosis (end-to-side).
- **Blalock–Taussig shunt (Modified).** Interposition graft between subclavian artery and uni- or bilateral pulmonary artery.
- **Waterston shunt.** Ascending aorta to main or right pulmonary artery (side-by-side).
- **Potts shunt.** Descending aorta to left pulmonary artery (side-by-side).
- **Central interposition tube graft**
- **Infundibular resection (Brock procedure) or closed pulmonary valvotomy**
- **Relief of right ventricular outflow tract obstruction without ventricular septal defect closure or with fenestrated VSD closure**

Shunts can usually be detected from suprasternal view. Color and continuous wave Doppler are usually very helpful for assessing the patency, tortuosity, and/or stenosis of the shunt. Magnetic resonance imaging (MRI) provides clearer images of the shunt (see Figure 7.4).

Assessment of pulmonary artery anatomy and pressure is mandatory at some point, in patients who have had previous palliation(s), because these shunts have inherent complications (distortion of the pulmonary arteries and

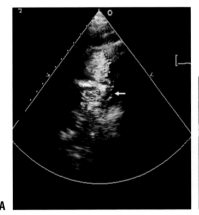
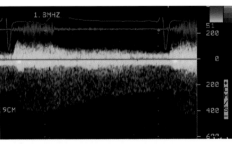

A   B

FIGURE 7.4. Suprasternal view from a patient with palliated tetralogy of Fallot with Blalock–Taussig shunt demonstrating patent shunt on (A) color flow Doppler and (B) continuous wave Doppler.

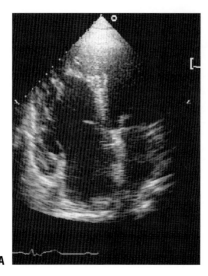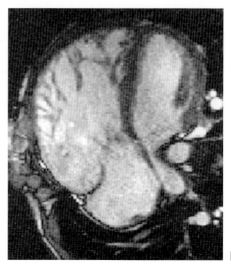

A   B

FIGURE 7.5. Apical four chamber view from a patient with repaired tetralogy of Fallot showing dilated right heart secondary to severe pulmonary regurgitation: (A) echocardiogram and (B) MRI.

development of pulmonary hypertension). Peripheral pulmonary artery stenosis, when present, may exacerbate pulmonary regurgitation, with its deleterious long-term effects on right ventricular function (see Figure 7.5).

Left ventricular dilatation and dysfunction may also develop secondary to volume overload. In patients with previous Brock procedure, residual right ventricular outflow tract obstruction, and significant pulmonary regurgitation can still be present (see Figure 7.6).

In view of the potential right-side complications in patients with unoperated or previously palliated tetralogy of Fallot, late repair should be considered in those suitable for surgery, which in turn should improve functional status and quality of life.

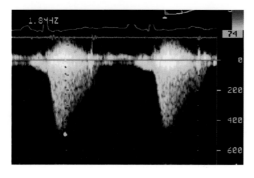

FIGURE 7.6. Continuous wave Doppler velocities across the right ventricular outflow tract from a patient with tetralogy of Fallot showing significant residual narrowing with a peak velocity of 5 m/s, equivalent to a pressure drop of 100 mm Hg.

7.1.2.3. Patients with Reparative Surgery

Reparative surgery for tetralogy of Fallot involves closing the ventricular septal defect and relieving the right ventricular outflow tract obstruction. The latter may involve pulmonary valvotomy; resection of infundibular muscle; right ventricular outflow tract patch or transannular patch (a patch across the pulmonary valve annulus); pulmonary implantation (homograft valve or other bioprosthesis); an extracardiac valved conduit placed between the right ventricle and the pulmonary artery, in patients with pulmonary atresia (congenital or acquired); or angioplasty/patch augmentation of central pulmonary arteries in patients with hypoplastic main pulmonary trunk and/or stenosis of the central pulmonary arteries.

Pulmonary regurgitation and right ventricular outflow tract obstruction are the most common residual hemodynamic lesions that contribute to the morbidity and mortality of these patients.

7.1.2.4. Assessment of Right Ventricular Outflow Tract

Parasternal short-axis or subcostal views are the best for studying right ventricular outflow tract. Two-dimensional images display the pulmonary valve and pulmonary artery anatomy and color and continuous wave Doppler confirm the level of stenosis, its severity, and pulmonary regurgitation.

7.1.2.4.1. Pulmonary Regurgitation

Pulmonary regurgitation can be quantified by using two criteria: jet diameter on color flow map and pulmonary regurgitation index.

- Jet diameter is measured at the pulmonary valve leaflets level during early diastole. Jet diameter >0.98 cm indicates significant regurgitation (see Figure 7.7).
- Pulmonary regurgitation index (PR index) is the ratio between pulmonary regurgitation time and total diastole. An index of <0.77 suggests severe pulmonary regurgitation.

From the pulmonary artery spectral Doppler, total diastolic time is measured as the time interval between the end of previous ejection to the beginning of the succeeding one. Pulmonary regurgitation time is measured from the onset of regurgitation to the end, when the regurgitation signal reaches the baseline (pressure equalization between pulmonary artery and right ventricle). The ratio of pulmonary regurgitation time to total diastole is taken as PR index. The lower the value, the more severe the regurgitation is (see Figure 7.8). Color jet diameter and pulmonary regurgitation index have been found to correlate closely with values of the pulmonary regurgitant fraction measured by MRI.

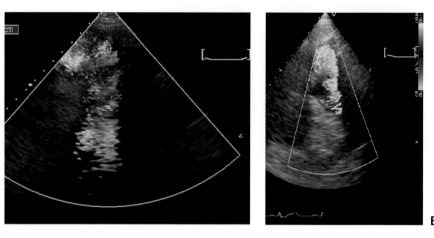

FIGURE 7.7. Parasternal short-axis view from two patients with tetralogy of Fallot and pulmonary regurgitation: (A) severe and (B) mild. Note the broad jet with lamina regurgitant flow in the patient with severe regurgitation.

7.1.2.4.1. Pulmonary Stenosis

Residual right ventricular afterload is also undesirable because of the increased risk of ventricular dysfunction and arrhythmia. Residual or progressive pulmonary stenosis after repair may occur at different levels. Incomplete resection of infundibula, small pulmonary artery annulus, or obstruction at pulmonary artery bifurcation or within proximal branches may result in right ventricular hypertension, followed by hypertrophy. Doppler criteria commonly used for the assessment of severity of right ventricular outflow tract obstruction are the same as those used for assessing isolated pulmonary valve stenosis.

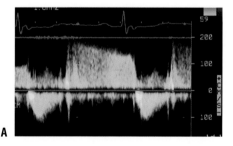
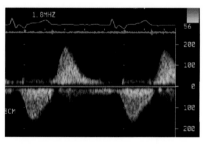

FIGURE 7.8. Continuous wave Doppler velocities of pulmonary regurgitation from two patients with tetralogy of Fallot demonstrating one with low PR index consistent with severe regurgitation (B) and the other with very long PR duration suggesting mild regurgitation (A).

- **Mild**. Pressure gradient <40 mm Hg, or right ventricular pressure <50% the left ventricular pressure.
- **Moderate**. Pressure gradient 40 to 70 mm Hg, or right ventricular pressure >50% the left ventricular pressure.
- **Severe**. Pressure gradient ≥70 mm Hg, or right ventricular pressure ≥ left ventricular pressure.

Severity of right ventricular outflow tract obstruction may be underestimated in the presence of right ventricular dysfunction and reduced stroke volume.

7.1.2.5. Assessment of the Right Ventricle

Assessment of the right ventricle includes assessment of its morphology (size and wall thickness) and function (systolic and diastolic). The former includes right ventricular inflow and outflow tracts. Right ventricular outflow tract is the region where the frequent presence of akinesis and aneurysmal formation contributes to ventricular dysfunction and predisposes to sustained ventricular tachycardia.

7.1.2.5.1. Right Ventricular Morphology

Right ventricular size can be measured from parasternal long-axis view, which represents right ventricular outflow dimension, and from the apical four chamber view by measuring right ventricular inlet diameter. Right ventricular outflow tract diameter >2.7 cm is compatible with increased end diastolic volumes by MRI. The literature also suggests that right ventricular inlet diameter >4 cm is consistent with cavity dilatation. Right ventricular outflow tract aneurysmal dilatation and akinetic patch area are best visualized from the parasternal short-axis view, and can be more clearly demonstrated by MRI (see Figure 7.9).

7.1.2.5.2. Right Ventricular Function

Right ventricular function has been known to be an echocardiographic challenge in part due to the complex geometry of the right ventricle.

- Routine measurement of right ventricular free wall long-axis excursion and myocardial tissue Doppler velocity are very useful in the follow up of these patients and can help monitoring the disease progress (see Figure 7.10).
- Antegrade diastolic flow detected by pulsed wave Doppler in the main pulmonary artery coinciding with atrial systole (*a* wave), presenting throughout the respiratory cycle, is a marker of right ventricular restrictive physiology. Retrograde flow during atrial systole can also be detected on superior and inferior vena cava flow (see Figure 7.11).

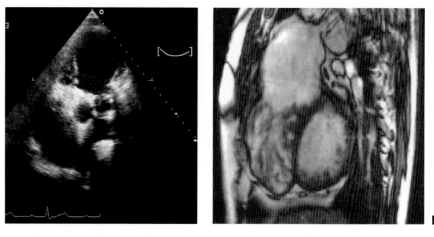

FIGURE 7.9. Parasternal short-axis view from a patient with repaired tetralogy of Fallot demonstrating aneurysmal and akinetic outflow tract: (A) echocardiogram and (B) MRI.

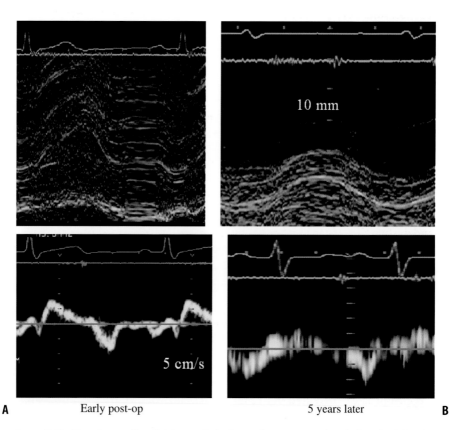

FIGURE 7.10. M-mode recording of right ventricular free wall movement and equivalent tissue Doppler velocities from a patient (A) soon after surgery and (B) 5 years later. Note the significant deterioration in ventricular function.

FIGURE 7.11. Continuous wave Doppler of pulmonary blood flow demonstrating late diastolic *a* wave (*arrow*) consistent with a stiff right ventricle.

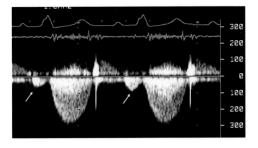

- Recently developed techniques of ultrasonic strain rate and strain indeces have been shown to detect and quantify regional wall motion abnormalities in repaired tetralogy of Fallot patients.
- Myocardial performance index (MPI) has been used to assess overall right ventricular performance.

MPI = (isovolumic contaction + isovolumic relaxation times)/ejection time

- Right ventricular dp/dt can also be measured from tricuspid regurgitation trace.
- Right ventricular end diastolic and end systolic volumes and ejection fraction derived from MRI are helpful in quantifying right ventricular systolic function.

7.1.2.5.3. Tricuspid Regurgitation

Tricuspid regurgitation may develop secondary to right ventricular dilatation and dysfunction. It can also be the consequence of surgical repair of ventricular septal defect. Severity of tricuspid regurgitation can be assessed from color flow mapping and continuous wave Doppler. From the continuous wave Doppler, velocity of tricuspid regurgitation pulmonary artery systolic pressure can be estimated using the equation

Pulmonary artery pressure = tricuspid regurgitation pressure drop + right atrial pressure (see Figure 7.12).

When tricuspid regurgitation is severe, the regurgitant flow velocity is reduced because of the raised right atrial pressure. The continuous wave Doppler profile of tricuspid regurgitant flow in this condition is more triangular in shape and ends so close to pulmonary valve closure sound (S2). Markedly reversed interventricular septal movement and dilatation of the right atrium are also present with severe tricuspid regurgitation (see Figure 7.13).

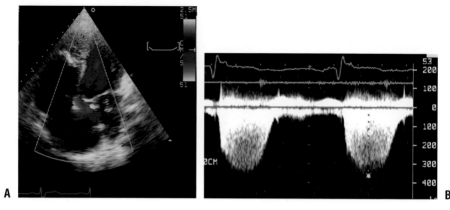

A   B

FIGURE 7.12. (A) Apical four chamber view from a patient with repaired tetralogy of Fallot showing dilated right heart with mild tricuspid regurgitation. (B) Continuous wave Doppler velocities of tricuspid valve regurgitation demonstrating a peak velocity of 3.5 m/s consistent with pressure drop of 50 mm Hg.

7.1.2.5.4. *Aortic Root Dimension and Aortic Regurgitation*

A subset of adult patients with repaired tetralogy of Fallot may present with ongoing aortic root dilatation that may result in aortic regurgitation. Furthermore, aortic root dilatation may predispose to aortic dissection and rupture. Therefore, aortic root size should be routinely assessed during follow up of tetralogy patients. The maximum diameter of the sinotubular junction at end diastole should be measured from M-mode trace using leading edge methodology taken from the parasternal long-axis view. From the same image, aortic root size is measured at three levels: hinge point, sinusus, and sinotubular junction (see Figure 7.14).

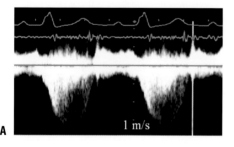
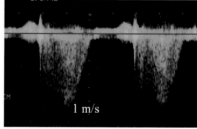

A   B

FIGURE 7.13. Continuous wave Doppler recordings from two patients, one with severe tricuspid regurgitation (A) and the other with mild regurgitation (B). Note the difference in the velocity profile, shape, and pressure drop.

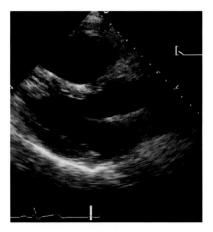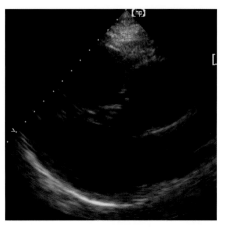

FIGURE 7.14. Left parasternal long-axis view from a patient with tetralogy of Fallot showing progressive aortic root dilatation over the course of 3 years.

Aortic root dilatation can be defined from the standard monograms for aortic root size at the sinotubular junction from normal adults, indexed to body surface area and age. Aortic root dilatation is taken as the ratio of observed to expected aortic root diameter >1.5.

Aortic valve regurgitation can be assessed using color flow Doppler and continuous wave Doppler. Color jet width measured during diastole, at the valve level of more than 10 mm, indicates significant regurgitation. Furthermore, when aortic-left ventricular pressure drop in end diastole is <40 mm Hg, it suggests significant regurgitation, particularly in patient with normal left ventricle end diastolic pressure (see Figure 7.15).

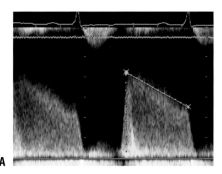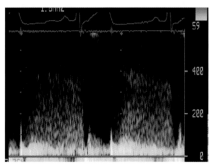

A   B

FIGURE 7.15. Continuous wave Doppler recording of aortic regurgitation from two patients, one with severe (A) and the other with mild (B). Note the significance fall in the aortic-left ventricular pressure drop in late diastole in the former.

7.1.2.5.5. Left Ventricular Diameter and Function

Left ventricular dilatation and dysfunction may relate to previous longstanding volume overload from left-to-right shunt due to palliative arterial shunts and also from chronic cyanosis, prior to repair. Left ventricular dysfunction may be secondary to acquired coronary artery disease as patients get older and such cavity dysfunction can be further exaggerated by aortic regurgitation. Ventricular interaction with right ventricular dysfunction is also present. Left ventricular dimensions can be measured from the parasternal long-axis view using M-mode recordings. Conventional methods for assessing left ventricular function (such as ejection fraction and fractional shortening) can be applied in the absence of severe aortic regurgitation.

7.1.2.5.6. Residual Shunt

Residual ventricular septal defects are common around the ventricular septal defect patch area. Ventruicular septal defect size and shunt velocity should always be assessed. From the shunt velocity, right ventricular pressure can be evaluated (see Figure 7.16).

Right ventricular systolic pressure = systolic blood pressure – left-to-right shunt pressure drop.

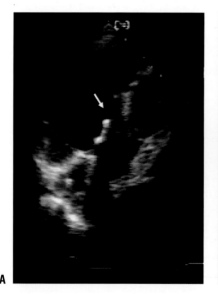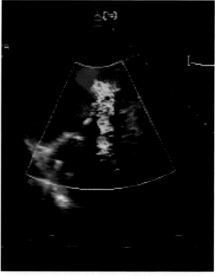

A   **B**

FIGURE 7.16. (A) Apical five chamber view showing residual ventricular septal defect (*arrow*) on two-dimensional image and (B) left-to-right shunt on color flow Doppler.

In the absence of right ventricular outflow tract obstruction and branch pulmonary artery stenosis, the right ventricular systolic pressure is similar to pulmonary artery systolic pressure. Occasionally, additional muscular ventricular septal defects can be present. Significant left-to-right shunt usually results in left atrial and left venticular volume overload and dilatation. Furthermore, shunts at atrial and arterial level can be seen. Significant left-to-right shunt at atrial level causes right atrial and right ventricular dilatation.

7.2. Pulmonary Atresia with Ventricular Septal Defect

This lesion is characterized by the absence of direct connection between the right ventricular chamber and the pulmonary arterial tree, and the presence of a large ventricular septal defect. Pulmonary atresia may be at the valve level or complete absence of the main pulmonary artery. Blood flow to the pulmonary circulation is through an alternative route such as a patent ductus arteriosus (so-called simple pulmonary atresia) or major aortopulmonary collateral arteries (MAPCAs). The latter is also known as complex pulmonary atresia, where central confluent pulmonary arteries are commonly absent.

Due to the complex and heterogeneous pulmonary artery anatomy, patients seen in adult congenital heart disease clinic can be divided into three groups:

Group 1: Native survivor without any surgical intervention.

Group 2: Palliated either by surgically created aortopulmonary shunts, unifocalization of collateral vessels or banding of large native aortopulmonary collateral vessels to prevent pulmonary arterial hypertension.

Group 3: Repaired by creating a connection between the right ventricle and the pulmonary artery using homograft or heterograft valved or nonvalved conduit and repair of intracardiac anomaly (such as closure of ventricular septal defect or repair of atrioventricular septal defect).

7.2.1. Native Survivals (Unrepaired)

The intracardiac anatomy is similar to unrepaired tetralogy of Fallot, except the absence of right ventricular outflow tract and forward flow from the right ventricle to the pulmonary artery. Parasternal images show the large subaortic ventricular septal defect with overriding aorta which is often dilated. However, the spectrum of intracardiac anatomy may also include abnormalities of atrioventricular and ventriculoarterial connections, such as atrioventricular septal defect, double outlet right ventricle, or transposition of the great arteries. The right ventricle is often hypertrophied due to pressure overload. When there is excessive pulmonary blood flow either from collaterals or aortopulmonary shunt, left ventricular dilatation occurs. Aortic root dilatation often results in variant degrees of aortic regurgitation. When it is severe, aortic regurgitation further increases the volume overload of the ventricles. Aortic valve stenosis from calcified valve has been seen in older survivors, which may be the result of longstanding large stroke volume. With ventricular dysfunction, the degree of aortic stenosis is often underestimated. Restrictive biventricular dysfunction demonstrated by large "*a*" wave on SVC and IVC flow and giant "*a*" wave on jugular venous pulse is often seen later in life. Suprasternal views are ideal for studying the aortopulmonary artery shunts or collateral flow. Normally the flow from the shunt is continuous during the cardiac cyrcle with higher velocity (about 4 m/s) during systole. Low velocity flow detected from the shunt or collateral vessels may indicate increased pulmonary artery pressure or raised resistance.

7.2.2. Repaired Patients

It is important to assess conduit function, which is often located anterior just behind the sternum. When the conduit is heavily calcified, it is difficult to demonstrate its anatomy by two-dimensional imaging, but color and continuous wave Doppler are helpful in detecting conduit patency. Turbulent flow on color and increased flow velocity on continuous wave Doppler suggest conduit stenosis. Due to the position of the conduit, continuous wave Doppler may not line up with the maximum velocity jet. Residual intracardiac shunt or aortopulmonary shunts are often seen in these patients, which not only contribute to the ventricular volume overload but are also the potential sites for infective endocarditis (see Figures 7.17 to 7.20).

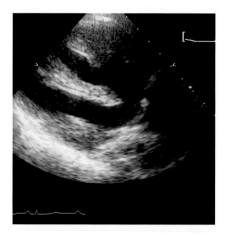

FIGURE 7.17. Parasternal view from an unrepaired patient showing a large subaortic ventricular septal defect and a dilated aortic root overriding the septum (>50%). Significant right ventricle hypertrophy also is seen in this view.

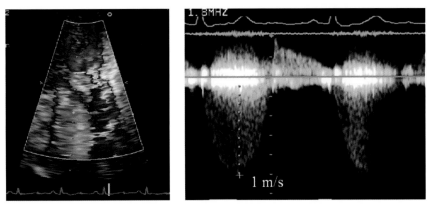

Figure 7.18. (A) Right ventricle to pulmonary artery conduit stenosis from a patient with repaired tetralogy of Fallot with an aortic homograft between the right ventricle and the pulmonary artery. Color flow shows turbulent flow across the valve and (B) continuous wave Doppler recorded peak velocity of 5 m/s across the valve.

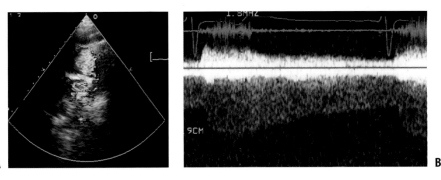

Figure 7.19. Suprasternal view showing shunt flow on (A) color flow Doppler and (B) continuous wave Doppler from a patient with previous Blalock–Taussig shunt.

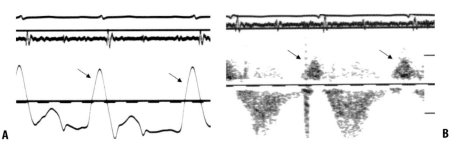

Figure 7.20. (A) SVC trace and (B) Doppler recording of flow from a patient with biventricular restrictive disease showing flow reversal in late diastole (*arrow*).

7.3. Transposition of the Great Arteries (Ventriculoarterial Discordance)

Sequential segmental analysis of the heart enables complex congenital cardiac malformations to be described in a straightforward and simple fashion. All hearts, normal or abnormal, are built from three segments: the atria, the ventricular mass, and the arterial trunks. Following this approach, after the diagnosis of situs (atrial arrangement) has been established, the mode of atrioventricular connection is determined.

7.3.1. Unoperated Transposition of Great Arteries

Transposition of great arteries describes the abnormal arrangement of the heart in which the morphological right atrium is connected to a morphological right ventricle which, in turn, gives rise to the aorta, while the morphologically left atrium is connected to morphologically left ventricle that supports the pulmonary trunk. The segmental connections, therefore, are concordant at atrioventricular junction, but discordant at ventriculoarterial junction. The hemodynamic consequence of complete transposition is parallel systemic and pulmonary circulations. When there is no additional abnormality, it is usually called simple transposition. Coexisting lesions, such as patent ductus arteriosus, large ventricular septal defect, pulmonary stenosis, or aortic coarctation, may also be present (complex transposition).

Ventriculoarterial connections and the relative size of the great arteries can be defined best from subcostal, parasternal, and apical views. Together with the subcostal view, the sagittal view identify the ventriculoarterial relationship in infants and small children. In both planes the transposed aorta usually arises from an anterior, right-side chamber of right ventricular morphology, while the transposed pulmonary artery arises from a posterior left-side chamber of left ventricular morphology. Subcostal coronal views are most useful to demonstrate the size of interatrial communication (see Figure 7.21).

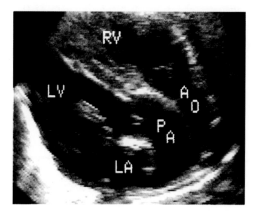

FIGURE 7.21. Parasternal view from a patient with transposition of great arteries showing the relationship between the great arteries and ventricles. Note the pulmonary artery arising from the morphological left ventricle and the aorta from the morphological right ventricle.

FIGURE 7.22. Parasternal short-axis view from a patient with transposition of great arteries showing double circle appearance of the two semilunar valves.

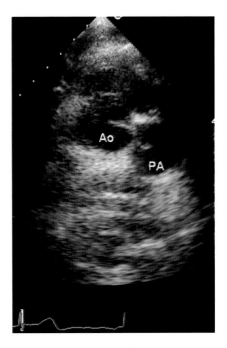

Parasternal long-axis view is very useful for displaying the ventriculoarterial connections and a number of abnormalities, such as subpulmonary stenosis, ventricular septal defect, and valvar stenosis.

Parasternal short-axis view displays the aortic and pulmonary root with the respective semilunar valves, the so-called double circle appearance due to the parallel position of the great arteries. Usually the aortic root lies anterior and to the right of the pulmonary root. The aorta and pulmonary arteries can be defined by their ranching pattern. Bifurcation of the pulmonary arteries is considered the morphologic hallmark for the pulmonary trunk. The coronary arteries are the diagnostic feature of the aortic root (see Figure 7.22).

Apical views are particularly useful for observing the relative size of the ventricles, ventricular function, and atrioventricular valve regurgitation by color flow and continuous wave Doppler, for the recognition of a wide variety of ventricular septal defects. Doppler techniques also help in assessing left ventricular outflow tract abnormalities and the size of branch pulmonary arteries.

Suprasternal imaging is important in defining associated arch abnormalities, the size of the pulmonary arteries, and the patency and size of the ductus arteriosus.

7.3.2. Transposition of Great Arteries Post Surgical Repair

The long-term problems that are associated with repaired transposition of great arteries depend on the type of repair. Three types of repair are well known.

The oldest patient have intra-atrial repair, either Mustard or Senning type. The relatively young patients have arterial switch operation. In patients with coexisting pulmonary stenosis, Rastelli type repair is usually performed.

In patients with Mustard or Senning repair, surgically created venous pathway stenosis is a common complication in the late follow up. This can be assessed by examining the superior and inferior vena cava flow into the atria using color and pulsed wave Doppler. Right (systemic) ventricular dysfunction and tricuspid regurgitation should also be assessed in all such patients. Other residual lesions, such as baffle leak, residual ventricular septal defect, dynamic subpulmonary stenosis, pulmonary hypertension due to pulmonary venous hypertension should all be investigated. In addition, patients with exertional symptoms; angina-like chest discomfort or breathlessness could be physiologically assessed by stress echocardiography. A recent study has shown close relationship between right ventricular function in these patients and exercise tolerance assessed by cardiopulmonary exercise testing. Furthermore, in these patients, the right ventricular function becomes very abnormal at fast heart rate, demonstrating disturbances similar to those seen in patients with coronary artery disease, suggesting a possible underlying ischemic dysfunction. These findings are consistent with those found in dilated cardiomyopathy (see Figures 7.23 to 7.29).

The arterial switch procedure seems to avoid a lot of the above-mentioned complications, provided supravalvar pulmonary stenosis and/or coronary Steal stenosis are the most common amongest them. Aortic valve (previous pulmonary valve) function should always be checked. These patients have the obvious advantage of using their left ventricle as the systemic ventricle. Conduit stenosis and/or regurgitation is a known complication in patients with Rastelli

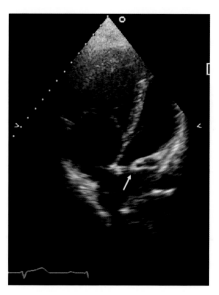

FIGURE 7.23. Apical four chamber view from a patient with transposition of great arteries post Mustard repair. A baffle has been shown within the atria to guide the pulmonary venous return to the morphological right ventricle.

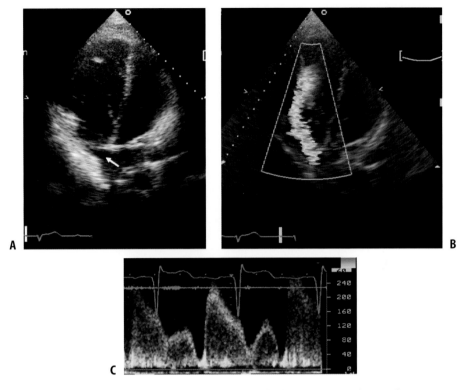

FIGURE 7.24. (A) Apical four chamber view showing narrowed pulmonary venous pathway at the entrance to the right atrium (*arrow*), (B) turbulent flow on color flow Doppler, and (C) increased flow velocity on pulse wave Doppler.

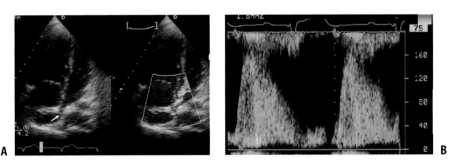

FIGURE 7.25. (A) Apical four chamber view shows narrowed SVC pathway with turbulent flow on color flow map and (B) increased flow velocity on pulse wave Doppler.

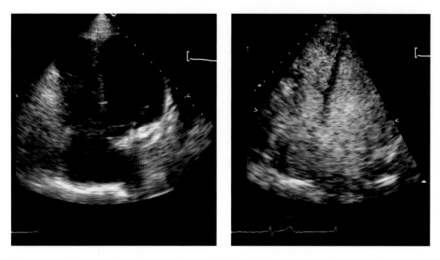

FIGURE 7.26. Contrast echocardiogram showing baffle leak. Contrast injected via a peripheral vein. It appears in both atria and ventricles at nearly the same time, suggesting blood mixing at the atrial level.

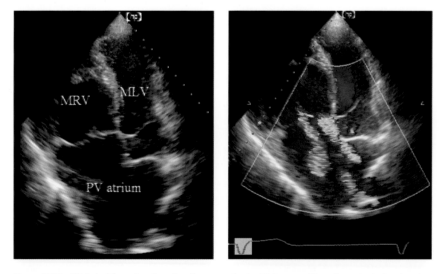

FIGURE 7.27. (A) Apical four chamber view from a patient with transposition of great arteries showing right ventricular and pulmonary venous atrial dilatation and (B) significant tricuspid regurgitation on color Doppler.

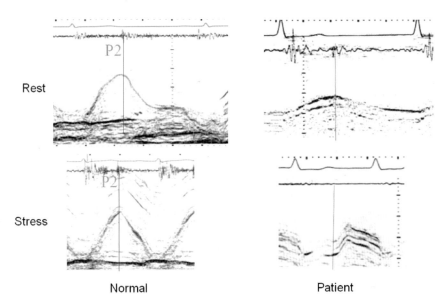

FIGURE 7.28. Right ventricular free wall M-mode at rest (top) and stress (bottom) from a normal control and a patient post Mustard repair showing stress induced incoordination in the patient (right) suggesting underlying ischemia.

type repair. The conduit is almost always difficult to visualize on two-dimensional images. Color and continuous wave Doppler help in confirming conduit lesions. From ticuspid regurgitation Doppler, right ventricular pressure can be assessed and indirectly assess conduit status (see Figure 7.30).

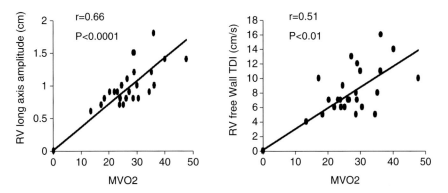

FIGURE 7.29. A graph showing a close relationship between right ventricular function and exercise MVO2 from a group of Mustard patients.

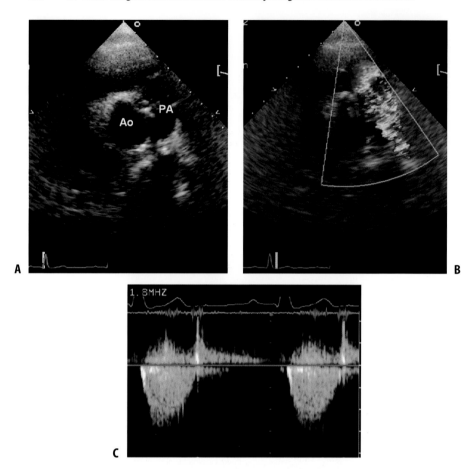

FIGURE 7.30. (A) Parasternal short-axis views from a patient with transposition of great arteries after arterial switch repair demonstrating important supravalvar pulmonary stenosis on two-dimensional, image, turbulent flow on (B) color flow Doppler, and (C) high velocity on continuous wave Doppler.

7.4. Eisenmenger Syndrome

Eisenmenger syndrome is defined as pulmonary hypertension associated with congenital heart disease with reversed or bidirectional shunting leading to chronic cyanosis. It matters very little where the shunt happens to be.

The simple and common lesions are large ventricular septal defect, patent ductus arteriosus, and atrial septal defect. Complex lesions without pulmonary outflow tract obstruction may also develop Eisenmenger physiology, such as atrioventricular septal defect, truncus arteriosus, aortopulmonary window, ventricular arterial discordance and atrioventricular and ventriculoarterial discordance with a nonrestrictive ventricular septal defect, and single ventricular type heart. The likelihood of developing pulmonary vascular disease depends on both the site and the size of the communication. Patients with a shunt at the aortopulmonary or ventricular level are more likely to develop Eisenmenger physiology than patients with a communication at atrial level. It may occur in patients with previous palliative surgery, such as surgically created arterial-to-pulmonary artery shunts (e.g., Potts and Waterston anastomoses), reparative surgery but with significant residual shunt, or sliding pulmonary banding. In a small number of patients, after radical repair for the shunt lesion, the pulmonary artery pressure can increase persistently until reaches systemic level.

Echocardiography assesses the basic anatomy and determines the level of systemic-to-pulmonary artery shunting. Two-dimensional images demonstrate the cardiac anatomy and defects, and color Doppler shows the shunt level and direction (see Figures 7.31 to 7.36).

Using continuous wave Doppler, pulmonary artery pressure can be assessed by the following flow velocity and equations.

1. Flow velocity across the intracardiac shunt:

$$PASP = BP - 4V^2$$

(PASP, pulmonary artery systolic pressure; BP, systolic blood pressure; V, maximum flow velocity across the shunt)

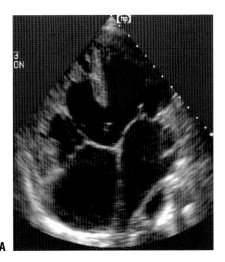
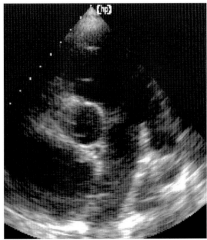

A   B

FIGURE 7.31. (A) Apical four chamber view showing a large perimembranous inlet ventricular septal defect. (B) Parasternal short-axis view showing dilated main pulmonary artery and branches suggesting significantly increased pulmonary arterial pressure.

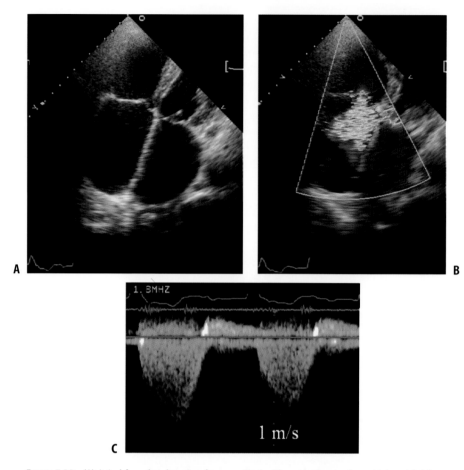

FIGURE 7.32. (A) Apical four chamber view from a patient with repaired secundum atrial septal defect; note thickened inter-atrial septum because of the patch repair. (B) Color Doppler showing moderate tricuspid regurgitation and (C) continuous wave Doppler showing a maximum velocity of 4 m/s suggest significantly increased pulmonary arterial pressure.

2. Tricuspid regurgitation velocity:

$$PASP = 4V^2 + RAP$$

(PASP, pulmonary artery systolic pressure; V, maximum flow velocity of tricuspid regurgitation; RAP, right atrial pressure)
3. Pulmonary regurgitation velocity (V):

$$MPAP = 4(V_{PR-PD})^2 + RAP$$

$$PAEDP = 4(V_{PR-ED})^2 + RAP$$

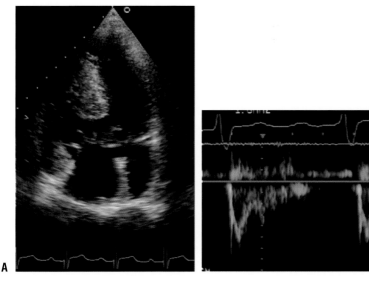

FIGURE 7.33. (A) Apical four chamber view from a patient with an atrioventricular septal defect; note significant right ventricular hypertrophy and dilated right atrium as a consequence of increased pulmonary arterial pressure. (B) Doppler flow across the pulmonary valve with very short acceleration time suggests increased pulmonary vascular vesistance.

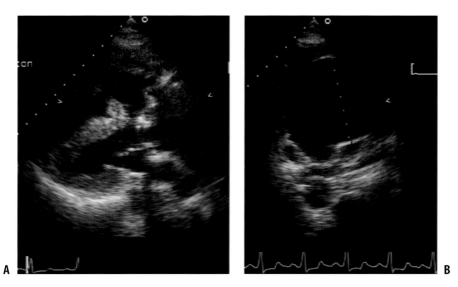

FIGURE 7.34. (A) Parasternal long-axis and (B) short-axis views from a patient with type I Truncus arteriosus; note right ventricular dilatation and hypertrophy on the long-axis view and markedly dilated main pulmonary artery on the short-axis view.

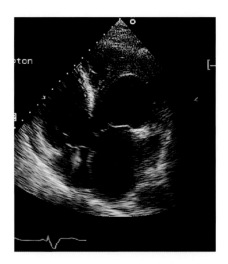

FIGURE 7.35. Apical four chamber view from a patient with atrioventricular and ventricular arterial discordance (CC-TGA) and ventricular septal defect; note the intraventricular septum is bulging towards left suggesting raised pulmonary ventricular pressure.

(MPAP, mean pulmonary artery pressure; V_{PR-PD}, peak pulmonary regurgitation velocity in early diastole; RAP, right atrial pressure; PAEDP, pulmonary artery end diastolic pressure; V_{PR-ED}, end diastolic velocity of pulmonary regurgitation)

In patients with Eisenmenger syndrome, ventricular function should be routinely assessed and the degree of pulmonary and tricuspid valve regurgitation documented. Right ventricular dysfunction may occur later in life in these

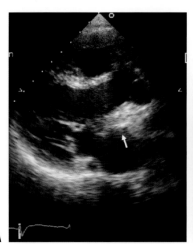
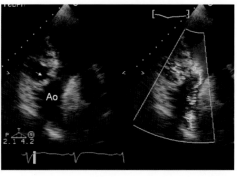

A

B

FIGURE 7.36. (A) Parasternal view from a patient with repaired double outlet right ventricle and residual ventricular septal defect; note the aorta and mitral valve discontinuity (*arrow*). (B) Apical five chamber view showing distance between the left ventricle and aorta and residual ventricular septal defect (*arrow*) at the previous patch with low velocity left-to-right shunt on color flow Doppler suggesting pulmonary arterial hypertension.

FIGURE 7.37. Significantly reduced right ventricular filling time due to long tricuspid regurgitation, which contributes to reduced right ventricular stroke volume.

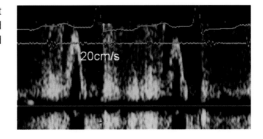

patients. However, their hearts more closely resemble normal fetal heart than the adult heart. Right and left ventricular wall thickness is nearly equal in patients with defects distal to the tricuspid valve and the interventricular septum is midline and flat throughout the cardiac cycle. The regression of right ventricular wall thickness may never occur and contractile function is long term preserved in the majority of patients. But actual filling time may become shortened due to diastolic dysfuction, which limits cardiac output, especially when heart rate increases.

The ventricles of these patients appear to function as a common unit with an almost linear relationship between systolic function of the two ventricles; when the right ventricle fails, the left does as well. The most common cause of death in patients with Eisenmenger syndrome is not heart failure or sudden cardiac death, but secondary to intrapulmonary hemorrhage or rupture of a dilated pulmonary trunk (see Figures 7.37 and 7.38).

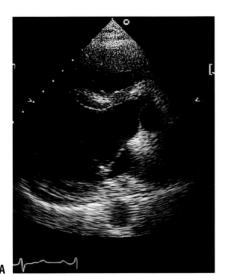
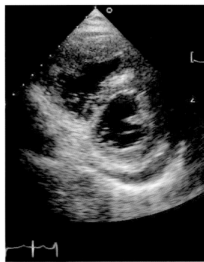

A   B

FIGURE 7.38. (A) Parasternal long-axis view from a patient with a ventricular septal defect who developed biventricular failure later in life; note dilated left ventricle with impaired ventricular function. (B) Parasternal short-axis view showing pericardial effusion.

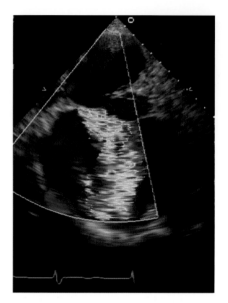

FIGURE 7.39. Modified parasternal short-axis view from a patient with previously repaired atrial septal defect showing severe tricuspid regurgitation on color flow Doppler.

Significant tricuspid and pulmonary valve regurgitation are often associated with clinical deterioration. In some cases, severely dilated pulmonary artery may dissect or have thrombus formation (see Figures 7.39 and 7.40).

Pericardial effusion may develop and it is often the sign of ventricular failure.

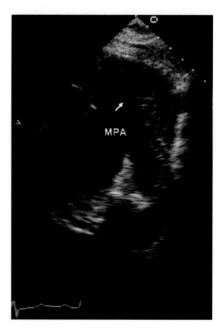

FIGURE 7.40. Parasternal short-axis view of main pulmonary artery and branches from a patient with Eisenmenger syndrome showing dissection of main pulmonary artery and thrombus formation (*arrow*).

7.5. Congenitally Corrected Transposition of Great Arteries

In congenitally corrected transposition of great arteries, the morphological right atrium is connected to the morphological left ventricle, which support the pulmonary trunk, while the left atrium is connected to the right ventricle, which gives rise to the aorta. Congenitally corrected transposition describes the discordant atrioventricular connections that are accompanied by discordant ventriculoarterial connection. In this condition, the morphologic left ventricle lies to the right and the morphologic right ventricle lies to the left in a side-to-side fashion. The great vessels connection can be appreciated from a variety of views, including the parasternal apical and subcostal. It is therefore important to define the ventricular morphology and atrioventricular and ventriculoarterial connection to diagnose the discordant atrioventricular connection. Distinction between the morphologically right and left ventricles is possible by their characteristic features. The most reliable echocardiographic features are the septal attachment of the right atrioventricular valve and the lack of ventricular septal attachment of the mitral valve. Other features for this condition are trabecular pattern (heavy course trabeculations) of the morphological right ventricle, ventricular shape, and the position of the atrioventricular valve attachment that can be seen in the apical and subcostal four chamber views and in parasternal short-axis view. Corrected transposition of great arteries is commonly associated with other cardiac malformations: ventricular septal defects, valvar or subvalvar pulmonary stenosis, and abnormalities of the left-side tricuspid valve. Ebstein anomaly of the left-side tricuspid valve can be identified and assessed echocardiographically. Coarctation of the aorta may also be encountered as an associated defect (see Figures 7.41 to 7.45). Finally, patients are predisposed to acquired complete heart block (risk of 2–3% per annum).

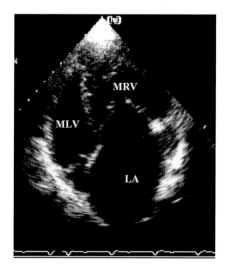

FIGURE 7.41. Apical four chamber view from a patient with congenitally corrected transposition of the great arteries (CC-TGA) showing the pattern of atrioventricular valve displacement and the characteristic trabeculation of the morphological right ventricle.

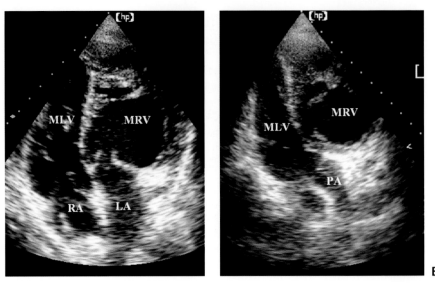

FIGURE 7.42. (A) Apical four chamber view from a patient with congenitally corrected transposition of the great arteries with ventricular septal defect. (B) Apical five chamber view showing the pulmonary artery arising from the morphological left ventricle.

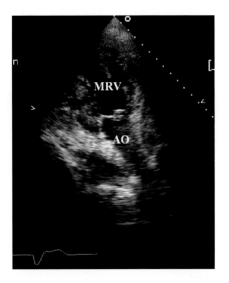

FIGURE 7.43. Apical view showing the aorta arising from a morphological right ventricle.

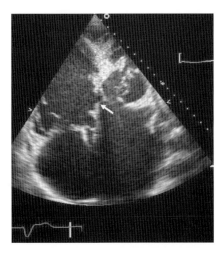

FIGURE 7.44. Apical four chamber view from a patient with CC-TGA, ventricular septal defect, and Ebstein anomaly of the tricuspid valve; note the marked apical displacement of septal leaflet of tricuspid valve (*arrow*).

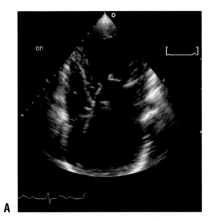
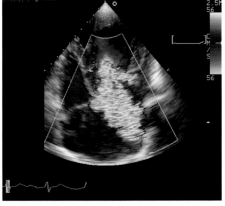

A   B

FIGURE 7.45. (A) Apical four chamber view of a patient with CC-TGA, systemic ventricular dysfunction, and (B) severe tricuspid regurgitation on color flow Doppler. Note the tricuspid valve is structurally normal but leaflets are not coapting, suggesting the regurgitation is functional.

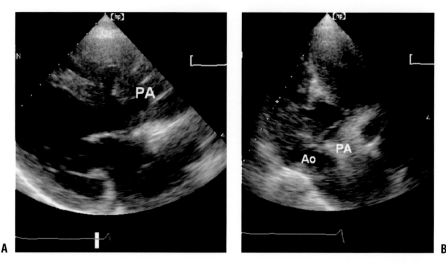

FIGURE 7.46. (A) Parasternal long-axis and (B) apical views from a patient with double outlet right ventricle and ventricular septal defect. Note the pulmonary artery is nearer to the ventricular septal defect.

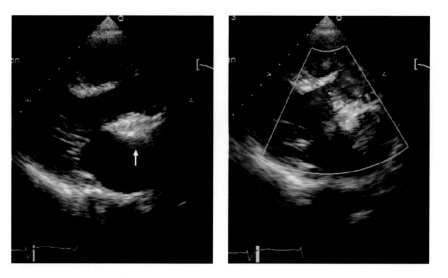

FIGURE 7.47. Parasternal view of a patient with double outlet right ventricle post Rastelli repair showing aorto-mitral valve discontinuity (*arrow*).

7.6. Double Outlet Right Ventricle

Double outlet right ventricle can be defined as more than half of the circumference of both arterial valves, irrespective of the nature of their supporting structures, are connected to the morphologically right ventricle (50% rule). The double outlet right ventricle can best be considered within a spectrum of conditions. In one spectrum lies the condition of double outlet right ventricle at one end and tetralogy of Fallot with subaortic ventricular septal defect at the other end. In another spectrum, the form of double outlet right ventricle associated with a subpulmonary ventricular septal defect (known as the Taussig–Bing anomaly) at one end and transposition of the great arteries with subpulmonary ventricular septal defect at the other end. A key feature of double outlet right ventricle is the position of the ventricular septal defect. Several positions have been described: a subaortic position; a subpulmonary position; doubly committed subarterial position; and a position distant from both great vessels, that is, a noncommitted ventricular septal defect (see Figures 7.46 and 7.47).

Parasternal long-axis views are best to evaluate the relationship of the vessels to each other and to the ventricular septal defect. When the ventricular septal defect is subaortic, the overriding has to be greater than 50% so as to distinguish it from tetralogy of Fallot. When the defect is subpulmonary, the differentiation is between double outlet right ventricle and transposition of great arteries with ventricular septal defect.

8
Univentricular Heart (Singe Ventricle)

8.1. Unoperated Univentricular Heart

The arrangement in which both atria connect to one ventricle is described as double inlet ventricle. Univentricular atrioventricular connection by means of an absent left or right connection is frequently referred to in the literature as mitral and tricuspid atresia. In most "univentricular hearts", there are two ventricular chambers with one major (dominant) ventricle and a second rudimentary chamber. The rudimentary ventricle is usually situated anteriorly either rightward or leftward and is more often of right ventricular morphology. The pulmonary artery usually arises posteriorly from the large main chamber, which frequently is of left ventricular morphology, whereas the aorta usually rises anteriorly from the rudimentary outlet chamber. Where the associated ventricular septal defect is small in this setting, it leads effectively to subaortic stenosis.

8.1.1. Double Inlet Ventricle

The echocardiographic hallmark of double inlet ventricle is more than 50% of both atrioventricular valves open into a single and large ventricle. This finding may be demonstrated from a variety of views, including parasternal, apical, and subcostal transducer locations (see Figures 8.1 and 8.2).

In an absent right atrioventricular connection (classical tricuspid atresia), the tricuspid atresia is usually an absent connection, but occasionally may be a valvar atresia.

In an absent left atrioventricular connection (mitral atresia), the morphology is essentially similar to that described in the classical tricuspid valve disease but involving the mitral valve. As the pulmonary venous return to the left atrium, there has to be always a communication at the atrial level for survival, although this may become restrictive with growth.

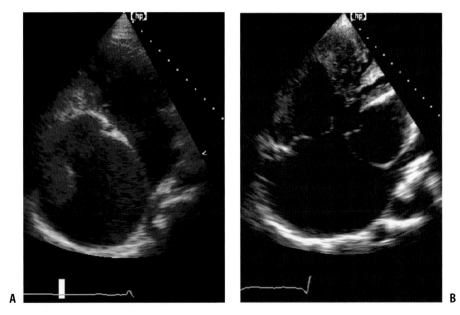

A

B

FIGURE 8.1. Apical views from two patients with univentricular hearts due to absent (A) right and (B) left atrioventricular connections.

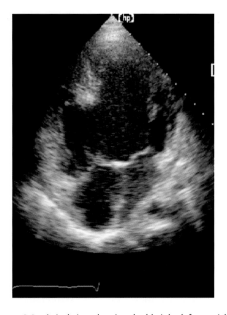

FIGURE 8.2. Apical view showing double inlet left ventricle.

8.1.2. Atrioventricular Valve Morphology and Function

Atrioventricular valve insufficiency in tricuspid atresia and other forms of univentricular atrioventricular connection are fairly common. Atrioventricular valve regurgitation is also a marker of adverse prognosis in double inlet ventricle. Valvar stenosis and obstruction proximal to the deformed atrioventricular valve, such as cor triatriatum or supravalvar mitral ring, although uncommon, may also be present (see Figure 8.3).

8.1.3. Ventricular Morphology and Function

The display of ventricular trabecular morphology can be considerably difficult to study by echocardiography. The orientation of the ventricular septum itself and the position of the rudimentary ventricle are commonly used for echocardiographic definition of ventricular morphology. Anterior rudimentary chambers are almost invariably of right ventricular morphology, whereas posterior rudimentary chambers are almost always of left ventricular morphology. When no outlet chamber is identified by echocardiography, the morphology of the

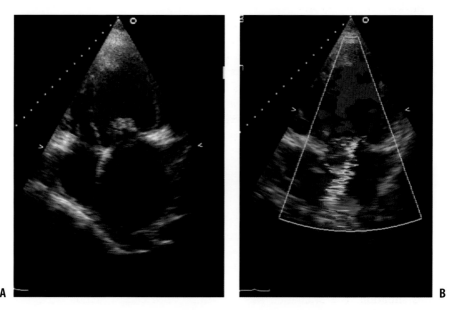

A   B

FIGURE 8.3. (A) Apical views from a patient with univentricular heart demonstrating thickened left atrioventricular valve and dilated left atrium. (B) Significant left atrioventricular valve regurgitation is shown on color flow Doppler.

ventricle may be regarded as indeterminate. Evaluation of the size and function of the main chamber provides prognostic information about the potential for success of the Fontan type procedure.

8.1.4. Position of the Outlet Chamber and the Size of the Interventricular Communication

A rudimentary right ventricle is always located anteriorly, superiorly, and to either the left or the right side. A rudimentary left ventricle is always located posteriorly. The interventricular communication may be restrictive initially or become restrictive with time. Color Doppler, pulsed, or continuous wave Doppler may help in assessing the severity of the restriction.

8.1.5. Great Vessel Position and Ventriculoarterial Connection

Abnormalities of ventriculoarterial connections are an integral part of hearts with a univentricular atrioventricular connection. The most frequent ventriculoarterial connection is discordance (transposed) with the pulmonary artery arising from the main chamber posteriorly and the aorta arising from the outlet chamber anteriorly. Imaging the vessels and their connection is best achieved from parasternal, apical, and subcostal views. In the classic form of double inlet ventricle, the pulmonary blood flow is either limited or excessive. When the pulmonary flow is limited, the obstruction may be at various sites from the subpulmonary area through to the supravalvar level. When there is excessive pulmonary blood flow, there is no obstruction (or very little) of flow to pulmonary artery; there is however, limited systemic flow. Concordant ventriculoarterial connection, where the pulmonary artery arises from a rudimentary right ventricle and the aorta arises from the main left ventricular chamber, is less common. Such a situation is referred to as the Holmes's heart. If atrial isomerism is present, abnormalities of pulmonary and systemic venous drainage occur frequently.

8.2. Postsurgical Palliation

Treatment of patients with single ventricle varies according to anatomy. Palliative procedures include a systemic–pulmonary artery shunt to increase pulmonary blood flow and pulmonary artery banding to limit pulmonary blood flow. In the modern era, Fontan type operation is the most definitive procedure in this situation. The evaluation should include ventricular function, atrioventricular valve function (stenosis or regurgitation), thrombus formation, functional status of either shunt or the Fontan circulation, and closure of the ventricular septal defect or bulb chamber.

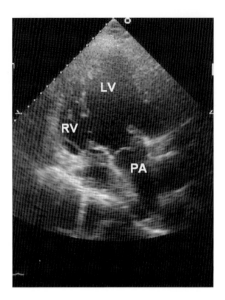

FIGURE 8.4. Apical views from a patient with univentricular heart showing the discordant ventriculoarterial connection.

8.2.1. Single Ventricle and Atrial Arrhythmia

Atrial arrhythmia is common in patients with single ventricles. The etiology of arrhythmia is likely to be multifactorial. Recent evidence suggests a distorted normal atrial electromechanical delay that allows the left atrium to contract before the right. Such extent of electromechanical disturbances may set a substrate for atrial arrhythmia, particularly atrial flutter (see Figure 8.4).

9
Congenital Anomalies of the Coronary Arteries

9.1. Ectopic Origin of the Coronary Artery from the Aorta

There is a considerable anatomical variety with these entities. The two most common patterns associated with actual or potential compromise of coronary artery flow and myocardial perfusion are:

1. Left coronary artery that arises aberrantly from the right sinus of Valsalva and passes between the aorta and right ventricular infundibulum.
2. Right coronary artery arising aberrantly from the left sinus of Valsalva and passes between the aorta and right ventricular infundibulum.

Echocardiography demonstrates the presence of ectopic coronary artery and its ostium, proximal course, and relationship to right ventricular outflow tract. When there is compromised coronary flow, stress echocardiogram can reveal myocardial regional wall motion abnormalities that would suggest ischemic dysfunction. In nonechogenic subjects, electron beam tomography or multislice computed tomography angiography may be the diagnostic tool of choice.

9.2. Anomalous Origin of the Left Coronary Artery from the Pulmonary Artery

This is a rare congenital anomaly where patients would die in infancy or early childhood without surgical intervention. Less than 10% of patients survive into adolescence or adulthood without intervention. In this anomaly, the left main coronary artery arises from the pulmonary trunk and then proceeds to the normal pattern of branching into left anterior descending and left circumflex arteries. Patients who survive into adult life usually develop intercoronary collateral circulation from normally perfused right coronary artery through myocardial collaterals to the anomalous left coronary system. Blood from the right coronary artery travels retrogradely through the left main coronary artery to the pulmonary trunk. Patients usually present with left ventricular dysfunction and mitral valve insufficiency secondary to the papillary muscle ischemic dysfunction.

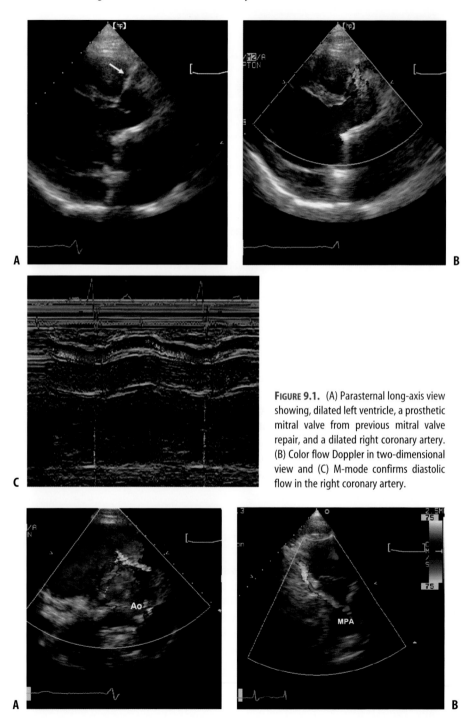

FIGURE 9.1. (A) Parasternal long-axis view showing, dilated left ventricle, a prosthetic mitral valve from previous mitral valve repair, and a dilated right coronary artery. (B) Color flow Doppler in two-dimensional view and (C) M-mode confirms diastolic flow in the right coronary artery.

FIGURE 9.2. (A) Parasternal short-axis view showing retrograde flow from the right coronary through (B) the left coronary artery into the pulmonary trunk.

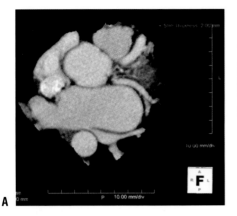
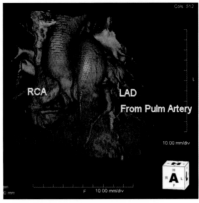

A

B

FIGURE 9.3. Electron beam tomography showing anomalous left coronary artery arising from the pulmonary trunk.

Echocardiography is an essential diagnostic tool for this condition. Parasternal long-axis view often shows the dilated and dysfunctional left ventricle. The mitral valve looks anatomically normal but functionally incompetent. Because the right coronary artery is often dilated in this condition, the proximal right coronary artery segment is easily seen in this view. Parasternal short-axis view confirms an absent origin of left coronary artery from the aortic root. Retrograde flow from the right coronary artery into the pulmonary trunk is easily seen with appropriate color gain settings. The dilated proximal right coronary artery can also be seen on this view. Collateral coronary artery flow within the myocardium may be demonstrated on color flow Doppler. Apical four chamber view shows dilated and dysfunctional left ventricle and/or wall motion abnormality and aneurysm formation, as well as functional mitral regurgitation (see Figures 9.1, 9.2, and 9.3).

9.3. Coronary Arteriovenous Fistula

In this condition, there is a fistulous communication of variable size between the coronary artery and, usually, a cardiac chamber. The proximal feeding coronary artery is usually aneurysmal and there is variable degree of obstruction at the distal site near the entrance of the receiving cardiac chamber. Fistulae originate more from the right coronary artery than the left. The proximal segment of the coronary arteries originates normally from the aorta. Most coronary fistulae enter the right atrium, but some enter the coronary sinus or the right ventricle.

9.3.1. Echocardiographic Examination

Parasternal long- and short-axis views are the best to demonstrate the dilated proximal coronary arteries. Depending on the chamber the fistula enters, parasternal short-axis and four chamber views usually reveal the abnormal flow into the right atrium, right ventricle, or coronary sinus. The flow from the fistula is usually continuous with high velocity during ventricular systole. When there is obstruction at the site of entrance, the high velocity occurs throughout the cardiac cycle.

Most adult patients with coronary arteriovenous fistula have a small shunt. There will be mild volume overloading on the receiving cardiac chamber. Myocardial ischemia from coronary steal is rare or mild at rest. Stress echocardiogram helps in demonstrating exercise-related myocardial ischemic changes which in turn assist in decision making. A large-size coronary fistula is usually treated surgically, whereas small ones can be occluded with coils (see Figure 9.4).

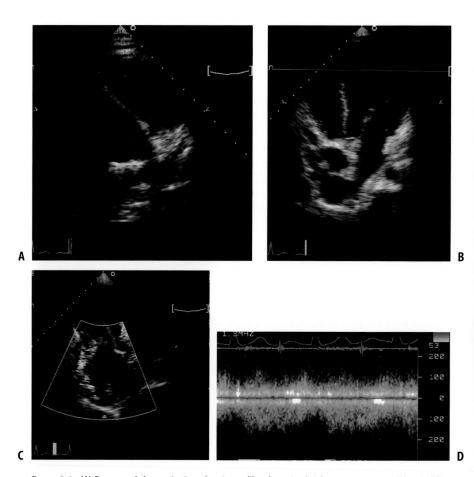

FIGURE 9.4. (A) Parasternal short-axis view showing a dilated proximal right coronary artery. (B) Apical five chamber view showing the right coronary artery entering into the right atrium, where (C) turbulent flow on color Doppler and (D) continuous flow with increased flow velocity suggests some degree of obstruction.

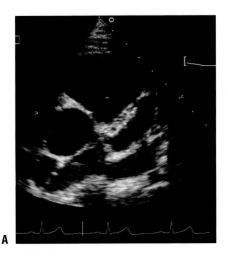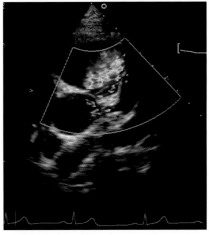

A   B

FIGURE 9.5. (A) Parasternal short-axis view shows left coronary artery aneurysm from a patient with previous Kawasaki disease. (B) Color flow Doppler shows turbulent flow in the proximal end of the left main coronary artery.

9.4. Coronary Artery Aneurysm (Kawasaki Disease)

Coronary artery aneurysms in adults are mostly the consequence of previous Kawasaki disease in early childhood. The aneurysms commonly involve the proximal segments of the coronary arteries with potential thrombotic occlusion. As a consequence, ischemic ventricular dysfunction occurs and there is the possibility of acute coronary syndrome (see Figure 9.5).

10
Infective Endocartidis

Nearly all adult patients with congenital heart disease (repaired, palliated, or unoperated) are at risk of infective endocarditis. Echocardiography plays an important role in the diagnosis and follow up of patients with endocarditis, and its unique high frame rate makes it ideal for detecting even small vegetations that could easily be missed by other noninvasive imaging techniques. Echocardiography also assists in clinical decision making, for example, surgical intervention during the treatment period. The most common lesions susceptible to superimposed infection, are those of the left ventricular outflow tract, which include subaortic stenosis, aortic valve disease, and post aortic valve replacement. The second high risk group of lesions are small unoperated ventricular septal defects and tetrology of Fallot.

The whole mark of infective endocarditis is the developement of vegetation, which is an oscillating intracardiac mass attached to a valve or to a supporting structure across the path of regurgitant jets, or on an implanted material (artificial valve) in the absence of an alternative anatomical explanation. Infective endocarditis may also occur at the site of a jet lesion, for example, around a small ventricular septal defect (see Figures 10.1 to 10.4).

Although common, vegetations are not by any means the only manifestations of infective endocarditis. Other complications are abscess formation, valve perforation, fistula formation, and partial dehiscence of prosthetic valves (see Figures 10.5, 10.6, and 10.7).

Infective endocarditis may affect lesions outside the heart, for example, surgically created shunts, coarctation sites, or collaterals. Echocardiography may be limited in confirming the exact site of infection. Other imaging modalities, such as magnetic resonance imaging (MRI), may be more sensitive in indirectly suggesting the presence of such infection by detecting new aneurysm formation, increase in the size of a poststenotic dilatation, or a change in the size of a shunt (see Figure 10.8).

Despite the great sensitivity of echocardiography in detecting evidence for endocarditis, the diagnosis remains based on microbiological and clinical evidence. Echocardiographic appearance of lupoid and thrombotic noninfective vegetations could be quite similar and difficult to distinguish from infective

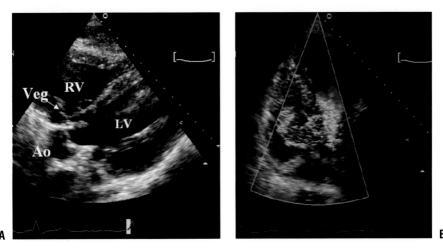

FIGURE 10.1. (A) Modified apical five chamber view shows a vegetation at the site of a small ventricular septal defect and (B) color flow Doppler with left-to-right shunt across the ventricular septal defect.

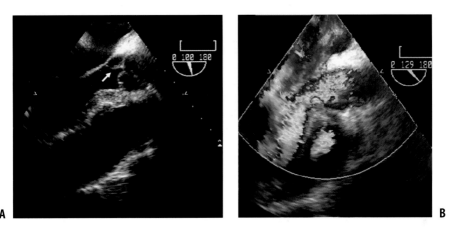

FIGURE 10.2. (A) Transesophageal echocardiogram of left ventricle outflow tract shows vegetation attached to a bicuspid aortic valve (*arrow*) and (B) severe aortic regurgitation on color flow Doppler.

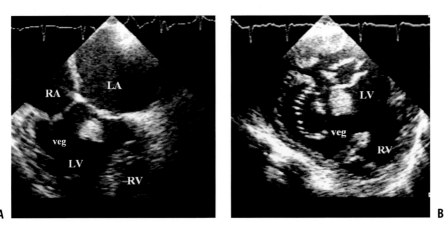

FIGURE 10.3. (A) Transesophageal echocardiogram four chamber view from a patient with double inlet left ventricle; note the large vegetation attached on the left atrioventricular valve. (B) Ventricular short-axis view shows clear anatomy of double inlet left ventricle and large vegetation on left atrioventriclular valve.

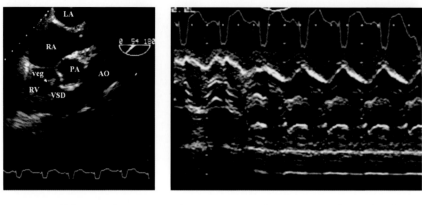

A   **B**

Figure 10.4. (A) Patient with transposition of great arteries. Note the vegetation attached on the right ventricle to pulmonary artery homograft valve. (B) M-mode recordings confirming the vegetation movement.

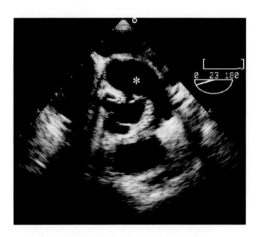

Figure 10.5. Transesophageal echocardiogram of aortic root from a patient with aortic root abscess after aortic valve replacement. Note the large cavity outside the aortic lumen (*).

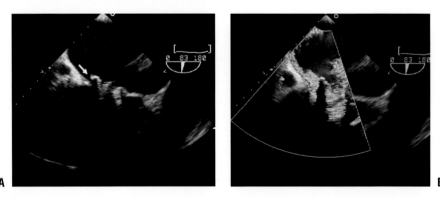

A   **B**

Figure 10.6. (A) Transesophageal echocardiogram from a patient with artificial mitral valve and clinical evidence for endocarditis shows the valve dehiscence (*arrow*) that caused (B) significant mitral regurgitation.

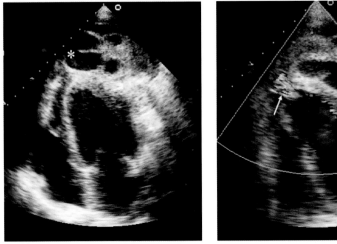

FIGURE 10.7. (A, B) Apical four chamber view from a patient with endocarditis complicated by left ventricle apex perforation (*arrow*) and abscess formation (*).

lesions. Healed vegetations after complete successful medical therapy may remain echocardiographically detectable for many years after an episode of endocarditis. Such vegetations should not be interpreted as evidence for recurrent infection unless there is supportive clinical and microbiological evidence.

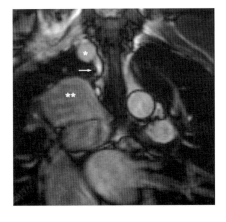

FIGURE 10.8. Magnetic resonance imaging scan from a patient with complex congenital heart disease and endocarditis on previous right Blalock–Taussig shunt (*arrow*). Note the infection at the shunt area causing large aneurysm formation (**).

11
Others

11.1. Myocarditis and Dilated Cardiomyopathy

Myocarditis and dilated cardiomyopathy may be seen in isolation in a structurally normal heart or in patients with congenital heart defects, before or after surgical repair. Differential diagnosis of the two conditions is echocardiographically difficult. It largely relies on the patient history, blood tests, and myocardial biopsy.

Echocardiographic features are similar in these two conditions, demonstrating globally impaired systolic left ventricular function irrespective of the cavity size. Toxic myocarditis, in particular, may present with normal left ventricular cavity size but very significantly impaired systolic function. An ideal example is the cardiotoxic effect of cancer chemotherapy, for examples, anthracycline. Some of these patients may recover after stopping the chemotherapy (see Figure 11.1).

Although rare, a small ventricular septal defect may be associated with a picture similar to dilated cardiomyopathy, with significant impairment of left ventricular function. Symptoms in this condition are usually disproportionate to the size of the ventricular septal defect in the absence of pulmonary hypertension. Closing the ventricular septal defect in this circumstances has been noted to be associated with recovery of left ventricular size and function.

Patients with Marfan syndrome may develop left ventricular cavity dilatation and impairment of systolic function, even in the absence of significant mitral or aortic valve dysfunction; this is a picture not different from dilated cardiomyopathy. The exact nature of myocardial disease in Marfan syndrome is not clearly understood.

11.2. Constrictive Pericarditis and Restrictive Cardiomyopathy

Constrictive pericarditis and restrictive cardiomyopathy are two completely different diseases but have similar clinical manifestations. The most common signs are those of fluid retention that is resistant to diuretics and raised venous

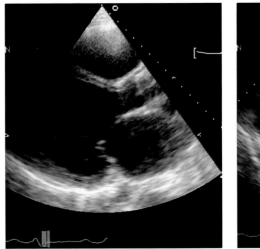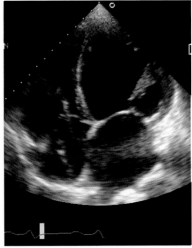

A B

Figure 11.1. (A) Parasternal long-axis and (B) apical four chamber views from a patient with dilated cardiomyopathy secondary to excess alcohol intake.

pressure. While constrictive pericarditis is a pathology that involves the pericardium, restrictive cardiomyopathy is a myocardial disease. The most common cause of constrictive pericarditis is tuberculosis, which is rarely seen. The most common cause of restrictive cardiomyopathy is the idiopathic type. In constrictive pericarditis, the heart may be anatomically completely normal, but in restrictive cardiomyopathy the characteristic features are normal ventricular cavity size with good systolic function, normal atrioventricular valve anatomy and function, but dilated right or left atrium. In this condition ventricular filling is always of the restrictive pattern, demonstrating short isovolumic relaxation time, short early diastolic "E" wave deceleration time, and small late diastolic "A" wave filling component. Patients with large left atrium are bound to develop atrial fibrillation; in them, the late diastolic filling component will be absent. Furthermore, because of ventricular myocardial stiffness, atrial systole fails to pump blood forward into the ventricular cavity resulting in retrograde flow in the vena cava or the pulmonary veins, which could easily be documented by pulsed wave Doppler (see Figures 11.2 and 11.3).

An additional characteristic feature of the two conditions is the pattern of the vena cava flow. Pericardial constriction limits the inward movement of the ventricular minor axis, making ventricular systole dependent on the atrioventicular ring movement, towards the apex in systole. This causes an increase in atrial cavity size, a drop in pressure, and a systolic filling component of the atrium equivalent to the "X" descent on the venous pulse. In contrast,

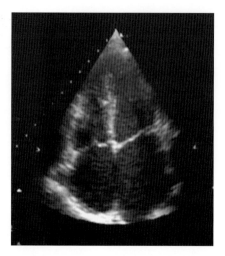

FIGURE 11.2. Apical four chamber view from a patient with fluid retention; note the normal ventricular size and large atria consistent with restrictive cardiomyopathy.

restrictive cardiomyopathy results in stiff ventricular myocardium and raised end diastolic pressure. This compromises late diastolic filling of the ventricle, making it almost entirely early diastolic in time. As a result, the rapid emptying of the atrium in early diastole allows atrial filling to take place almost entirely at the same time equivalent to the "Y" descent on the venous pulse.

It is always advisable to use more than one sign before deciding on the final diagnosis of these difficult conditions because management of the two conditions is completely different. While surgical pericardiectomy is recommended for patients with pericardial constriction, only diuretics and vasodilators may help in controlling patient symptoms in restrictive cardiomyopathy (see Figure 11.4).

A rare postoperative condition has recently been described as *pericardial restriction*. In patients who present with fluid retention long after open heart

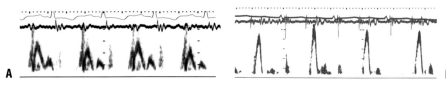

FIGURE 11.3. Left ventricular filling from two patients: one with constrictive pericarditis (A) and the other restrictive cardiomyopathy (B) demonstrating restrictive pattern in the patient with restrictive cardiomyopathy and a normal pattern in patient with constrictive pericarditis.

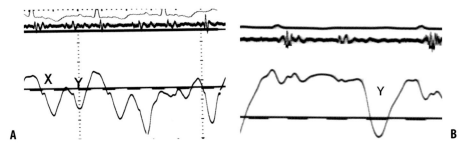

FIGURE 11.4. Venous pulse from patients with (A) constrictive pericarditis and (B) restrictive cardiomy-opathy demonstrating dominant X descent in constriction and Y descent in restriction.

surgery in whom diuretics are of limited benefit, detailed assessment of cardiac physiology to rule out pericardial restriction is needed. In these patients, the calcific pericardial disease involved the epicardium (the outermost layer of the myocardium). Because it is myocardial in origin, it presents with restrictive physiology in the same way as restrictive cardiomyopathy. The pericardium itself is involved in the pathological process but the predominant physiology is restriction. If symptomatic control with diuretics fails, pericardiectomy remains the only unexhausted option.

11.3. Ideopathic Pulmonary Arterial Hypertension

Ideopathic pulmonary arterial hypertension is a progressive disease which if untreated carries poor prognosis. Doppler echocardiography is a key screening and diagnostic tool for this condition. It not only provides an estimate of pulmonary artery pressure at rest and during exercise, but it also excludes any secondary causes for pulmonary hypertension, predicts prognosis, and monitors the response to therapeutic interventions.

The gold standard definition of pulmonary arterial hypertension is based on the measurement of mean pulmonary arterial pressure at cardiac catheterization. Pulmonary arterial hypertension is confirmed when the mean pulmonary artery pressure at rest is 25 mm Hg or 30 mm Hg on exercise. According to the World Health Organization, an echocardiographic diagnosis of mild pulmonary hypertension is systolic pulmonary artery pressure of 40 to 50 mm Hg, which corresponds to tricuspid regurgitation velocity on Doppler echocardiography of 3.0 to 3.5 m/s. There is no absolute cutoff value for the diagnosis of pulmonary hypertension by echocardiography.

Patients with normal resting pulmonary artery pressure but exertional dyspnea and clinical suspicion for raised pulmonary artery pressure, exercise/stress echocardiography may be used for monitoring changes in pulmonary artery pressure during exercise, thus differentiating physiological from pathological pulmonary hypertension. Normally there is mild increase in pulmonary artery pressure with exercise, but well-conditioned athletes are capable of increasing the systolic pulmonary artery pressure to 60 mm Hg with exercise. High stroke volume and cardiac output contribute to this phenomenon.

11.3.1. Assessing the Severity of Pulmonary Hypertension

11.3.1.1. Right Ventricular Size and Function

Because of the chronic right ventricular pressure overload, most patients present with enlarged right-side chambers, right ventricular hypertrophy, and reduced global right ventricle systolic function. Right ventricular dimensions, shape, and wall thickness can all be assessed from two-dimensional echocardiographic images. Right ventricular end diastolic dimension can be measured from M-mode parasternal long-axis view and right ventricular inflow dimension can be obtained from apical four chamber view just below the tricuspid valve.

Right ventricular end diastolic area (RV-EDA) and end systolic cavity area (RV-ESA) are conventionally determined by planimetry technique and tracing the endocardial border in the apical four chamber view in the plane of the mitral and tricuspid valve. The use of cavity contrast agents may improve the accuracy of the technique.

Right ventricular function can be assessed using the following parameters:

1. Right ventricular percentage change in area: this can be calculated as: $100 \times (RVEDA - RVESA)/RVEDA$.

2. Right ventricular long-axis function: This can be obtained by placing the M-mode cursor across the right atrioventricular junction from apical four chamber view. From these recordings, long-axis amplitude is directly measured as well as the time intervals.

3. Long-axis velocities in systole and diastole can easily be obtained using Tissue Doppler Imaging technique, particularly of the right ventricular free wall.

4. Myocardial Performance Index (Tei index): This index represents the ratio between the sum of the isovolumic contraction time and isovolumic relaxation time with respect to ejection time. This ratio has been found to correlate with $-dp/dt$, thus it is believed to provide a global assessment of the overall ventricular performance. The right ventricular performance index is relatively unaffected by heart rate, right ventricular pressures, or the severity of tricuspid regurgitation. It has good reproducibility and is particularly useful for the follow up of patients with established diagnosis. Right ventricular ejection time itself has been shown to improve with appropriate treatment in patients with pulmonary arterial hypertension (see Figure 11.5.)

FIGURE 11.5. Apical four chamber view from a patient with pulmonary hypertension showing dilated right-side chambers with a thickened right ventricular wall.

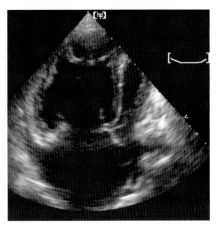

11.3.1.2. Interventricular Septal Shift

As pulmonary hypertension progresses, and pulmonary artery pressure increases, significantly deformed septal adaptation occurs with the septum functioning as part of the right ventricle rather than the left ventricle. This results in asynchronous septal motion, which has its implications on early diastolic tension development in the left ventricle and, consequently, on the pattern of left ventricular filling, being mainly late diastolic in timing. A characteristic D-shaped left ventricle is a diagnostic feature for significant pulmonary hypertension. This can easily be detected from the parasternal short-axis view. With further progression of pulmonary hypertension, the septal flattening becomes frank deviation into the left ventricle, giving it a banana-shaped appearance. To assess the degree of septal deformity, the eccentricity index is used to measure the septal shift from the parasternal short-axis view at the level of the chordae tendinae. It is the ratio of the left ventricular minor axis parallel to the septum divided by the minor axis perpendicular to the septum, at end diastole and end systole. In normal subjects, the index is approximately 1, but in pulmonary hypertension it is significantly more than 1 at both end diastole and end systole (see Figure 11.6).

Late cases of pulmonary hypertension may present with signs and symptoms of right heart failure, particularly resistant fluid retention. In them, right ventricular systolic function (from long-axis amplitude) is grossly depressed and the pattern of right ventricular filling may show evidence for raised right atrial pressure. The right atrium is always dilated at this stage of disease. In primary pulmonary hypertension, the presence of pericardial effusion is a manifestation of right ventricular failure and very high right atrial pressure. Pericardial effusion has been shown in several studies to predict a poor outcome.

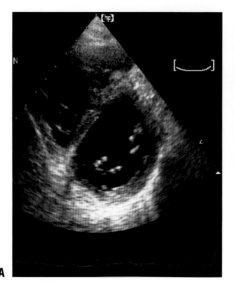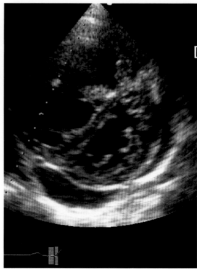

A   B

FIGURE 11.6. Parasternal short-axis view from two patients: (A) one with moderate and (B) the other with severe pulmonary hypertension. Note the banana-shaped left ventricular cavity in the latter compared with the D-shaped cavity in the former.

11.3.1.3. Right Atrial Area

This can be measured by planimetry in the apical four chamber view at end systole.

11.3.1.4. Patent Foramen Ovale

In patients with severe pulmonary hypertension, a left-to-right shunt through a patent foramen ovale is not easily seen on transthoracic echocardiography because of equalization of pressures between the two atria. The shunt is often right to left at certain periods of the cardiac cycle.

The presence of a patent foramen ovale or a small atrial septal defect can decompress high right-side pressures. Although patients may be mildly cyanosed, their cardiac output may be better than those without a shunt. Atrial septostomy may improve outcome in patients with severe pulmonary hypertension especially those with syncope.

For the estimation of pulmonary artery pressure by tricuspid regurgitation and pulmonary artery Doppler, please see Chapter 7, Eisenmenger syndrome.

Further Reading

Alboliras ET, Lombardo S, Antillon J. Truncus arteriosus with double aortic arch: two-dimensional and color flow Doppler echocardiographic diagnosis. Am Heart J 1995;129:415–417.

Daniel WG, Mügge A. Transesophageal echocardiography. N Engl J Med 1995;332: 1268–1279.

Driscoll DJ. Left-to-right shunt lesions. Pediatr Clin North Am 1999;46(2):355–68, x.

Fogel MA, Rychik J. Right ventricular function in congenital heart disease: pressure and volume overload lesions. Prog Cardiovasc Dis 1998;40:343–356.

Gatzoulis MA, Daubeney PEF, Webb GD. Diagnosis and management of adult congenital heart disease. Edinburgh: Churchill Livingstone; 2003.

Geva T, Gajarski RJ. Echocardiographic diagnosis of type B interruption of a right aortic arch. Am Heart J 1995;129:1042–1045.

Henein M, Sheppard M, Pepper J, et al. Clinical echocardiography. New York: Springer; 2004.

Hirsch R, Kilner P, Connelly M, et al. Diagnosis in adolescents and adults with congenital heart disease. Prospective assessment of individual and combined roles of magnetic resonance imaging and transesophageal echocardiography. Circulation 1994;90:2937–2951.

Ho S, McCarthy KP, Josen M, et al. Anatomic-echocardiographic correlates: an introduction to normal and congenitally malformed hearts. Heart 2001;86(Suppl 2): II3–II11.

Houston A, Hillis S, Lilley S, et al. Echocardiography in adult congenital heart disease. Heart 1998;80(Suppl 1):S12–S26.

Li W, Davlouros PA, Kilner PJ, et al. Doppler-echocardiographic assessment of pulmonary regurgitation in adults with repaired tetralogy of Fallot: comparison with cardiovascular magnetic resonance imaging. Am Heart J 2004;147:165–172.

Li W, Hornung TS, Francis DP, et al. Relation of biventricular function quantified by stress echocardiography to cardiopulmonary exercise capacity in adults with Mustard (atrial switch) procedure for transposition of the great arteries. Circulation 2004;110:1380–1386.

Li W, Sarubbi B, Sutton R, et al. Atrial and ventricular electromechanical function in 1-ventricle hearts: influence of atrial flutter and Fontan procedure. J Am Soc Echocardiogr 2001;14:186–193.

Masani ND. Transoesophageal echocardiography in adult congenital heart disease. Heart 2001;86(Suppl 2):II30–II40.

Muhiudeen Russell IA, Miller-Hance WC, Silverman NH. Intraoperative transesopha-geal echocardiography for pediatric patients with congenital heart disease. Anesth Analg 1998;87:1058–1076.

Pignatelli R, McMahon C, Chung T, et al. Role of echocardiography versus MRI for the diagnosis of congenital heart disease. Curr Opin Cardiol 2003;18:357–365.

Reddy SC, Chopra PS, Rao PS. Mixed-type total anomalous pulmonary venous connec-tion: echocardiographic limitations and angiographic advantages. Am Heart J 1995; 129:1034–1038.

Reddy SC, Chopra PS, Rao PS. Aneurysm of the membranous ventricular septum result-ing in pulmonary outflow tract obstruction in congenitally corrected transposition of the great arteries. Am Heart J 1997;133:112–119.

Rigby ML. Transoesophageal echocardiography during interventional cardiac catheteri-sation in congenital heart disease. Heart 2001;86(Suppl 2):II23–II29.

Russell IA, Rouine-Rapp K, Stratmann G, et al. Congenital heart disease in the adult: a review with internet-accessible transesophageal echocardiographic images. Anesth Analg 2006;102:694–723.

Sengupta PP, Khandheria BK. Transoesophageal echocardiography. Heart 2005;91: 541–547.

Seward J, Belohlavek M, O'Leary P, et al. Congenital heart disease: wide-field, three-dimensional, and four-dimensional ultrasound imaging. Am J Cardiac Imaging 1995; 9:38–43.

Silverman NH, McElhinney DB. Which two ventricles cannot be used for a biventricular repair? Echocardiographic assessment. Ann Thorac Surg 1998;66:634–640.

Silverman NH, McElhinney DB. Atrioventricular valve dysfunction: evaluation by Doppler and cross-sectional ultrasound. Ann Thorac Surg 1998;66:653–658.

Simpson I, Sahn D. Adult congenital heart disease: use of transthoracic echocardiography versus magnetic resonance imaging scanning. Am J Cardiac Imaging 1995;9:29–37.

Therrien J, Henein MY, Li W, et al. Right ventricular long axis function in adults and children with Ebstein's malformation. Int J Cardiol 2000;73:243–249.

Tworetzky W, McElhinney D, Brook M, et al. Echocardiographic diagnosis alone for the complete repair of major congenital heart defects. Am Coll Cardiol Found 1999; 33:228–233.

Wood MJ, Picard MH. Utility of echocardiography in the evaluation of individuals with cardiomyopathy. Heart 2004;90:707–712.

Bibliography

Diagnosis and Management of Adult Congenital Heart Disease by
Michael A. Gatzoulis, Gary D. Webb, Piers Daubeney. Churchill Livingstone; 2003
This practical resource provides essential guidance on the anatomic issues, clinical presentation, diagnosis and clinical management of adults with congenital heart disease. Each consistently structured, disease-oriented chapter discusses incidence, genetics, morphology, presentation, investigation and imaging, treatment and intervention. A wealth of illustrations, including line drawings, EKGs, radiographs and echocardiograms clearly depict the clinical manifestations of congenital defects.

Congenital Heart Disease in Adults by Joseph K. Perloff, John S. Child. W B Saunders; 2nd edition 1998
Clinical reference for cardiologists. Perloff and Child's book provides excellent clinical information on the special needs and concerns faced in caring for adults with congenital heart disease. First textbook of its kind in the field.

Congenital Heart Disease Adult by Welton M. Gersony, Marlon, S. Rosenbaum, Myron L. Weisfeldt. McGraw-Hill Professional; 2001
This guide to the broad spectrum of congenital heart defects helps to optimize adult patient care.

Congenital Heart Disease in Adults: A Practical Guide by Andrew Redington, Darryl Shore, Paul Oldershaw. W B Saunders; 1997
Concise text for cardiologists and family practitioners on the special aspects of managing congenital heart disease in adults. Takes the approach that these adults can't be treated as large children with congenital disease.

Cardiac Surgery by Nicholas Kouchoukos, Eugene Blackstone, Donald Doty, Frank Hanley, Robert Karp. W B Saunders; 3rd edition 2003
Essential textbook in both adult and pediatric cardiac surgery, updated and revised in a new, third edition. It thoroughly covers the full range of new and classic surgical procedures and presents the up-to-date clinical evidence practitioners need to make effective management decisions.

Moss and Adams' Heart Disease in Infants, Children, and Adolescents: Including the Fetus and Young Adult by Hugh D. Allen, Howard P. Gutgesell, Edward B. Clark, David J. Driscoll. Lippincott Williams & Wilkins; 6th edition 2000
Updated throughout, the sixth edition of Moss and Adams continues to be the primary cardiology text for those who care for infants, children, adolescents, young adults, and fetuses with heart disease. A comprehensive text covering basic science theory through clinical practice of cardiovascular disease in the young, this edition includes an expanded special section on young adults and a greatly expanded genetics section.

Color Atlas of Congenital Heart Disease: Morphologic and Clinical Correlation by Sew Yen Ho, E.J. Baker, M.L. Rigby, R.H. Anderson. Mosby; 1994
A correlation of the clinical and pathological features of congenital heart disease, including anatomy, imaging and pathology. This work covers all aspects of structural defects of the heart and major vessels arising during the development of the fetus, as well as conditions seen in neonates and young children. It provides a comprehensive review of incidence and actuality of various conditions, their characteristic features as defined by a range of investigative techniques, and detailed discussion of underlying pathology.

Paediatric Cardiology by Robert Anderson, E. Baker, M. Rigby, E. Shinebourne, M. Tynan. Churchill Livingstone; 2nd edition 2003
A comprehensive and exhaustive reference of fundamental and clinical aspects of heart disease in infancy and childhood. The contributors are well-known experts in the field and the editors are a world-class group who have published extensively in the field. Provides an up-to-date and authoritative account of pediatric cardiovascular fields covering embryology, morphology, pathophysiology, specific clinical conditions, treatments and the psychosocial aspects of caring for patients with heart disease.

Cardiac Arrhythmias after Surgery for Congenital Heart Disease by S. Balaji, P.C. Gillette, C.L. Case. Hodder Arnold; 2001
This comprehensive text discusses all aspects of atrial and ventricular cardiac arrhythmias in patients undergoing cardiac surgery for congenital heart problems. This area is one of growing interest, as an increasing number of individuals with heart defects live longer due to improved therapy, and are now facing new problems. The numbers and types of problems being tackled by invasive ablation techniques have been growing dramatically since the mid-1980s, and this publication aims to tie together the aspects of these conditions. Appropriate management of these patients critically depends on knowledge of the type of surgery, the types of arrhythmias these patients are prone to, and the therapeutic modalities that can be used to treat them.

"Congenital Heart Disease in Adults" by Judith Therrien and Gary D. Webb. In *Heart Disease: A Textbook of Cardiovascular Medicine*, 6th edition. Edited by Eugene Braunwald, Douglas P. Zipes, Peter Libby. Saunders; 2001
The essential *Textbook of Cardiovascular Medicine*, bringing cutting-edge advances in the field. Ninety-eight world authorities synthesize everything from the newest findings in molecular biology and genetics to the latest imaging modalities, interventional procedures and medications. The two adult congenital heart editors Drs Therrien and Webb in this latest edition encompass all of today's essential knowledge in the field.

Task Force on the Management of Cardiovascular Diseases During Pregnancy of the European Society of Cardiology
Expert consensus document on management of cardiovascular diseases during pregnancy. *European Heart Journal*, 2003, **24**, 761–781.

Canadian Cardiovascular Society Consensus Conference 2001 update
Can J Cardiol **2001** Sep; 17: 940–59; *Can J Cardiol* **2001** Oct; 17: 1029–50; *Can J Cardiol* **2001** Nov; 17: 1135–58.

Task Force on the Management of Grown Up Congenital Heart Disease of the European Society of Cardiology
Eur Heart J **2003, 24,** 1035–84.

Glossary

Prepared for the CCS Consensus Conference 2001 update: Recommendations for the Management of Adults with Congenital Heart Disease, published in *Canadian Journal of Cardiology* 2001; 17(9); 943ff. and accessible online at: http://www.ccs.ca/society/conferences/archives/2001/glossary.cfm and http://www.achd-library.com

Prepared by Jack M. Colman MD, FRCPC, FACC, Erwin Oechslin MD, FESC, and Dylan Taylor MD, FRCPC, FACC.

From *The ACHD Textbook: Diagnosis and Management of Adult Congenital Heart Disease* (eds MA Gatzoulis, GD Webb & P Daubeney) Philadelphia, PA: Churchill Livingstone, 2003.
Correspondence:
Jack M. Colman MD
Toronto Congenital Cardiac Centre for Adults at the Toronto General Hospital/UHN 1603–600 University Avenue Toronto ON M5G 1X5

The purpose of this glossary is to help guide those reading and researching in the area of adult congenital heart disease. It is meant to be a living document, constantly under revision, improvement, correction, as you, its users, find ways to ease the path for those who follow. To this end, if you cannot find a term you think should be here, or if you disagree with a definition, or see a way to improve it, drop us an e-mail before you move on. We promise to consider all feedback carefully, and to make additions and revisions on the website (http://www. achd-library.com/) often. We hope you fi nd the glossary helpful.
Jack Colman: j.colman@utoronto.ca
Erwin Oechslin: erwin.oechslin@usz.ch
Dylan Taylor: dtaylor@cha.ab.ca

Acknowledgment: we recognize with gratitude the ongoing contribution of Dr Robert Freedom, who generously agreed to review the work. We appreciate his support and encouragement.

aberrant innominate artery
A rare abnormality associated with right aortic arch wherein the sequence of arteries arising from the aortic arch is: right carotid artery, right subclavian artery, then (left) innominate artery. The latter passes behind the esophagus. This is in contrast to the general rule that the first arch artery gives rise to the carotid artery contralateral to the side of the aortic arch (i.e. right carotid artery in left aortic arch and left carotid artery in right aortic arch). *syn.* retro-esophageal innominate artery.

aberrant subclavian artery
The right subclavian artery arises from the aorta distal to the left subclavian artery. Left aortic arch with (retroesophageal) aberrant right subclavian artery is the most common aortic arch anomaly, first described in 1735 by Hunauld, and occurring in 0.5% of the general population.

absent pulmonary valve syndrome
Pulmonary valvular tissue is absent, resulting in pulmonary regurgitation. This rare anomaly uncommonly may be isolated; or it may be associated with ventricular septal defect, obstructed pulmonary valve annulus and massive dilatation and distortion of the pulmonary arteries. Absent pulmonary valve may also occur in association with other simple or complex congenital heart lesions.

ACHD
Adult congenital heart disease.

Alagille syndrome
see arteriohepatic dysplasia.

ALCAPA
Anomalous left coronary artery arising from the pulmonary artery. *see* Bland-White-Garland syndrome.

ambiguus
With reference to cardiac situs, neither right- nor left-sided (indeterminate). *see* situs.

Amplatzer® device
A self-centering device delivered percutaneously by catheter for closure of an atrial septal defect, a patent foramen ovale or a patent ductus arteriosus.

anomalous pulmonary venous connection
Pulmonary venous return to the right heart, which may be total or partial.

• total anomalous pulmonary venous connection (TAPVC). All pulmonary veins connect to the right side of the heart, either directly or via venous tributaries. The connection may be supradiaphragmatic, usually via a vertical vein to the innominate vein or the superior vena cava (SVC). The connection may also be infradiaphragmatic via a descending vein to the portal vein, the inferior vena cava (IVC) or one of its tributaries. Pulmonary venous obstruction is common in supradiaphragmatic connection, and almost universal in infradiaphragmatic connection.

- partial anomalous pulmonary venous connection (PAPVC). One or more but not all the pulmonary veins connect to the right atrium directly, or via a vena cava. This anomaly is frequently associated with sinus venosus atrial septal defect. *see also* scimitar syndrome.

aortic arch anomalies
Abnormalities of the aortic arch and its branching. Note that left or right aortic arch is defined by the mainstem bronchus that is crossed by the descending thoracic aorta and does not refer to the side of the midline on which the aorta descends.

In left aortic arch (normal anatomic arrangement) the descending thoracic aorta crosses over the left mainstem bronchus; the innominate artery branching into the right carotid and right subclavian artery arises first, the left carotid artery second and the left subclavian artery third. Usually, the first aortic arch vessel gives rise to the carotid artery that is opposite to the side of the aortic arch (i.e. the right carotid artery in left aortic arch and the left carotid artery in right aortic arch). The most important anomalies are:

- *abnormal left aortic arch*
  - left aortic arch with minor branching anomalies;
  - left aortic arch with retroesophageal right subclavian artery.
- *right aortic arch.* In right aortic arch the descending thoracic aorta crosses the right mainstem bronchus. It is often associated with tetralogy of Fallot, pulmonary atresia, truncus arteriosus and other cono-truncal anomalies. Types of right aortic arch branching include:
  - mirror image branching (left innominate artery, right carotid artery, right subclavian artery);
  - retroesophageal left (aberrant) subclavian artery with a normal calibre. Sequence of branching: left carotid artery, right carotid artery, right subclavian artery, then left subclavian artery;
  - retroesophageal diverticulum of Kommerell. *see* diverticulum of Kommerell;
  - right aortic arch with left descending aorta, i.e. retroesophageal segment of right aortic arch. The descending aortic arch crosses the midline toward the left by a retroesophageal route;
  - isolation of contralateral arch vessels: an aortic arch vessel arises from the pulmonary artery via the ductus arteriosus without connection to the aorta. This anomaly is very uncommon. Isolation of the left subclavian artery is the most common form.

- *cervical aortic arch.* The arch is located above the level of the clavicle.
- *double aortic arch.* Both right and left aortic arches are present, i.e. the ascending aorta splits into two limbs encircling the trachea and esophagus. The two limbs join to form a single descending aorta. There are several forms such as widely open right and left arches or hypoplasia/atresia of one arch (usually the left). This anomaly is commonly associated with patent ductus arteriosus. Double aortic arch creates a vascular ring around the trachea and the esophagus. *see also* vascular ring.
- *persistent 5th aortic arch.* Double-lumen aortic arch with both lumina on the same side of the trachea. Degree of lumen patency varies from full patency of both lumina to complete atresia of one of them. Seen in some patients with coarctation of the aorta or interruption of the aortic arch.
- *interrupted aortic arch.* Complete discontinuation between the ascending and descending thoracic aorta.
  - Type A: interruption distal to the subclavian artery that is ipsilateral to the second carotid artery.
  - Type B: interruption between second carotid artery and ipsilateral subclavian artery.
  - Interruption between carotid arteries.

aortic-left ventricular defect (tunnel)
Vascular connection between the aorta and the left ventricle resulting in left ventricular volume overload due to regurgitation from the aorta via the tunnel to the left ventricle.

aortic override
see tetralogy of Fallot.

aortic valve-sparing ascending aortic replacement
see David operation.

aorto-pulmonary collateral
Abnormal arterial vessel arising from the aorta, providing blood supply to the pulmonary arteries. May be single or multiple, and small or large (see also MAPCA). May be associated with tetralogy of Fallot, pulmonary atresia or other complex cyanotic congenital heart disease.

aorto-pulmonary septal defect
see aorto-pulmonary window.

aorto-pulmonary window
A congenital connection between the ascending aorta and main pulmonary artery, which may be contiguous with the semi-lunar valves, or, less often, separated from them. Simulates the physiology of a large PDA, but requires a more demanding repair. *syn.* aorto-pulmonary septal defect.

arterial switch operation
see Jatene procedure.

arteriohepatic dysplasia
An autosomal dominant multisystem syndrome consisting of intrahepatic cholestasis, characteristic facies, butterfly-like vertebral anomalies and varying degrees of peripheral pulmonary artery stenoses or diffuse hypoplasia of the pulmonary artery and its branches. Associated with microdeletion in chromosome 20p. *syn.* Alagille syndrome.

asplenia syndrome
see isomerism/right isomerism.

atresia, atretic
Imperforate, used with reference to an orifice, valve, or vessel.

atrial septal defect (ASD)
an inter-atrial communication, classified according to its location relative to the oval fossa (fossa ovalis):

- coronary sinus ASD. Inferior and anterior location at the anticipated site of the orifice of the coronary sinus. May be part of a complex anomaly including absence of the coronary sinus and a persistent left superior vena cava.
- ostium primum ASD. Part of the spectrum of atrioventricular septal defect (AVSD). Located anterior and inferior to the oval fossa such that there is no atrial septal tissue between the lower edge of the defect and the atrioventricular valves that are located on the same plane; almost always associated with a "cleft" in the "anterior mitral leaflet". This cleft is actually the separation between the leftsided portions of the primitive antero-superior and postero-inferior bridging leaflets. *see also* AVSD.
- ostium secundum ASD. Located at the level of the oval fossa.
- sinus venosus ASD. *see* sinus venosus defect.

atrial switch procedure
A procedure to redirect venous return to the contralateral ventricle. When used in complete transposition of the great arteries (either the Mustard or the Senning procedure) this accomplishes physiologic correction of the circulation, while leaving the right ventricle to support the systemic circulation. In patients with l-transposition of the great arteries and in patients who have had a previous Mustard or Senning procedure, it is used as part of a "double switch procedure" which results in anatomic correction of the circulation, with the left ventricle supporting the systemic circulation. *see also* double switch procedure.

atrioventricular concordance
see concordant atrioventricular connections.

atrioventricular discordance
see discordant atrioventricular connections.

atrioventricular septal defect (AVSD)
A group of anomalies resulting from a deficiency of the atrioventricular septum which have in common: 1) a common atrioventricular junction with a common fibrous ring, and a unique, 5-leaflet, atrioventricular valve; 2) unwedging of the aorta from its usual position deeply wedged between the mitral and tricuspid valves; 3) a narrowed subaortic outflow tract; 4) disproportion between the inlet and outlet portions of the ventricular septum. Echocardiographic recognition is aided by the observation that "left" and "right" AV valves are located in the same anatomic plane. Included in this group of conditions are anomalies previously known as (and often still described as) ostium primum ASD (partial AVSD), "cleft" anterior mitral and/or septal tricuspid valve leaflet, inlet VSD, and complete AVSD ("complete AV canal defect"). An older, obsolete, term describing such a defect is "endocardial cushion defect". *see also* endocardial cushion defect.

atrioventricular septum
The atrioventricular septum separates the left ventricular inlet from the right atrium. It has two parts: a muscular portion which exists because the attachment of the septal leaflet of the tricuspid valve is more towards the apex of the ventricle than the corresponding attachment of the mitral valve, and a fibrous portion superior to the attachment of the septal leaflet of the tricuspid valve. This latter portion separates the right atrium from the sub-aortic left ventricular outflow tract. *see also* Gerbode defect.

atrioventricular valve (AV valve)
A valve guarding the inlet to a ventricle. AV valves correspond with their respective ventricles, the tricuspid valve always associated with the right ventricle, and the mitral valve with the left ventricle. However, in the setting of an atrioventricular septal defect, there is neither a true mitral nor a true tricuspid valve. Rather, in severe forms there is a single atrioventricular orifice, guarded by a 5-leaflet AV valve. The "left AV valve" comprises the left lateral leaflet and the left portions of the superior (anterior) and inferior (posterior) bridging leaflets, while the "right AV valve" comprises the right inferior leaflet, the right antero-superior leaflet, and the right portions of the superior and inferior bridging leaflets.

• cleft AV valve. A defect often involving the left AV valve in AVSD formed by the conjunction of the superior and inferior bridging leaflets. A cleft may also be seen in the septal tricuspid leaflet. A similar but morphogenetically distinct entity may involve the anterior or rarely posterior leaflet of the mitral valve in otherwise normal hearts.

- common AV valve. Describes a 5-leaflet AV valve in complete AVSD that is related to both ventricles.
- overriding AV valve. Describes an AV valve that empties into both ventricles. It overrides the interventricular septum above a VSD.
- straddling AV valve. Describes an AV valve with anomalous insertion of tendinous cords or papillary muscles into the contralateral ventricle (VSD required).

autograft
Tissue or organ transplanted to a new site within the same individual.

AV septal defect (AVSD)
see atrioventricular septal defect (AVSD).

AV valve
see atrioventricular valve.

azygos continuation of the inferior vena cava
An anomaly of systemic venous connections wherein the inferior vena cava (IVC) is interrupted distal to its passage through the liver, and IVC flow reaches the right atrium through an enlarged azygos vein connecting the IVC to the superior vena cava. Usually, only hepatic venous flow reaches the right atrium from below. *see also* isomerism.

Baffes operation
Anastomosis of the right pulmonary veins to the right atrium (RA) and the IVC to the left atrium (LA) by using an allograft aortic tube to connect the IVC and the LA. (Baffes TG. A new method for surgical correction of transposition of the aorta and pulmonary artery. *Surg Gynecol Obstet* 1956, **102**, 227–233). This operation provided partial physiologic correction in patients with complete TGA. Lillehei and Varco originally described such a procedure in 1953. (Lillehei CW, Varco RL. Certain physiologic, pathologic, and surgical features of complete transposition of great vessels. *Surgery* 1953, **34**, 376–400.)

baffle
A structure surgically created to divert blood flow. For instance, in atrial switch operations for complete transposition of the great vessels, an intra-atrial baffle is constructed to divert systemic venous return across the mitral valve, thence to the left ventricle and pulmonary artery, and pulmonary venous return across the tricuspid valve, thence to the right ventricle and aorta. *see also* Mustard procedure. *see also* Senning procedure.

balanced
As in "balanced circulation", e.g. in the setting of VSD and pulmonary stenosis. The pulmonary stenosis is such that there is neither excessive pulmonary blood

flow (which might lead to pulmonary hypertension) nor inadequate pulmonary blood flow (which might lead to marked cyanosis). *see also* ventricular imbalance.

Bentall procedure

Replacement of the ascending aorta and the aortic valve with a composite graftvalve device and reimplantation of the coronary ostia into the sides of the conduit. (Bentall H, DeBono A. A technique for complete replacement of the ascending aorta. *Thorax* 1968, **23**, 338–339.)

- Exclusion technique: the native aorta is resected and replaced by the prosthetic graft.
- Inclusion technique: the walls of the native aorta are wrapped around the graft so that the prosthetic material is "included".

bicuspid aortic valve

An anomaly wherein the aortic valve is comprised of only two cusps instead of the usual three. There is often a raphe or aborted commissure dividing the larger cusp anatomically but not functionally. This anomaly is seen in 2% of the general population and in 75% of patents with aortic coarctation.

bidirectional cavopulmonary anastomosis

see Glenn shunt/bidirectional Glenn.

Björk modification

see Fontan procedure/RA-RV Fontan.

Blalock-Hanlon atrial septectomy

A palliative procedure to improve arterial oxygen saturation in patients with complete transposition of the great arteries, first described in 1950. A surgical atrial septectomy is accomplished through a right lateral thoracotomy, excising the posterior aspect of the interatrial septum to provide mixing of systemic and pulmonary venous return at the atrial level. (Blalock A, Hanlon CR. Surgical treatment of complete transposition of aorta and pulmonary artery. *Surg Gynecol Obstet* 1950, **90**, 1–15.)

Blalock-Taussig shunt

A palliative operation for the purpose of increasing pulmonary blood flow, hence systemic oxygen saturation. It involves creating an anastomosis between a subclavian artery and the ipsilateral pulmonary artery either directly with an end-to-side anastomosis (classical) or using an interposition tube graft (modified). (Blalock A, Taussig HB. The surgical treatment of malformations of the heart in which there is pulmonary stenosis or pulmonary atresia. *Journal of the American Medical Association* 1945, **128**, 189–202.)

Bland-White-Garland Syndrome
The left main coronary artery arises from the main pulmonary artery. The first
report describing clinical and pathologic features was published in 1933. (Bland
EF, White PD, Garland J. Congenital anomalies of the coronary arteries: report
of an unusual case associated with cardiac hypertrophy. *American Heart
Journal* 1933, **8**, 787; 801) *syn.* ALCAPA.

bridging leaflets
The superior and the inferior bridging leaflets of the AV valve are two leaflets
uniquely found in association with AVSD. They "bridge", or pass across, the
interventricular septum. When the central part of the bridging leaflet tissue
runs within the interventricular septum, the AV valve is functionally separated
into left and right components. When the bridging leaflets do not run within
the interventricular septum, but pass over its crest, a common AV valve guarding a common AV orifice (with an obligatory VSD) is the result.

Brock procedure
A palliative operation to increase pulmonary blood flow and reduce right-to-
left shunting in tetralogy of Fallot. It involved resection of part of the right
ventricle (RV) infundibulum using a punch or biopsy-like instrument intro-
duced through the right ventricle so as to reduce RV outflow tract
obstruction, without VSD closure. The operation was performed without
cardiopulmonary bypass. (Brock RC. Pulmonary valvotomy for the relief of
congenital pulmonary stenosis: report of three cases. *British Medical Journal*
1948, **1**, 1121–1126.)

bulbo-ventricular foramen
syn. primary foramen, primary ventricular foramen, primary interventricular
foramen. An embryological term describing the connection between the left-
sided inflow segments (primitive atrium and presumptive left ventricle) and
the right-sided outflow segments (presumptive right ventricle and cono-
truncus) in the primitive heart tube.

CACH (Canadian Adult Congenital Heart) Network
A co-operative nationwide association of Canadian cardiologists, cardiac sur-
geons and others, many of whom are situated in regional referral centers for
adult congenital heart disease, dedicated to improving the care of ACHD
patients. For more information, visit http://www.cachnet.org.

cardiac position
Position of the heart in the chest with regard to its location, and the orientation
of its apex.

• cardiac location—location of the heart in the chest:
  – levoposition—to the left;

- mesoposition—central;
- dextroposition—to the right.

Cardiac location is affected by many factors including underlying cardiac malformation, abnormalities of mediastinal and thoracic structures, tumors, kyphoscoliosis, abnormalities of the diaphragm.

- cardiac orientation—the base to apex orientation of the heart:
  - levocardia—apex directed to the left of the midline;
  - mesocardia—apex oriented inferiorly in the midline;
  - dextrocardia—apex directed to the right of the midline.

The base to apex axis of the heart is defined by the alignment of the ventricles and is independent of cardiac situs (sidedness). This axis is best described by echocardiography using the apical and subcostal 4-chamber views.

- cardiac sidedness. *see* situs.

cardiopulmonary study
A rest and stress study of cardiopulmonary physiology, including at least the following elements: resting pulmonary function, stress study to assess maximum workload, maximum oxygen uptake (MVO_2), anerobic threshold (AT), and oxygen saturation with effort.

Cardio-Seal® device
A device delivered percutaneously by catheter for closure of an ASD or PFO.

CATCH 22
Syndrome due to microdeletion at chromosome 22q11 resulting in a wide clinical spectrum. CATCH stands for **C**ardiac defect, **A**bnormal facies, **T**hymic hypoplasia, **C**left palate, and **H**ypocalcemia. Cardiac defects include conotruncal defects such as interrupted aortic arch, tetralogy of Fallot, truncus arteriosus, and double outlet right ventricle. *see also* DiGeorge syndrome, velocardio-facial syndrome.

cat's eye syndrome
A syndrome due to a tandem duplication of chromosome 22q or an isodicentric chromosome 22 such that the critical region 22pter—>q11 is duplicated. Phenotypic features include mental deficiency, anal and renal malformations, hypertelorism and others. Total anomalous pulmonary venous return is the commonest congenital cardiac lesion (in up to 40% of patients).

CHARGE association
This anomaly is characterized by the presence of coloboma or choanal atresia and three of the following defects: congenital heart disease, nervous system anomaly or mental retardation, genital abnormalities, ear abnormality or

deafness. If coloboma and choanal atresia are both present, only two of the additional (minor) abnormalities are needed for diagnosis. Congenital heart defects seen in the CHARGE association are: tetralogy of Fallot with or without other cardiac defects, atrioventricular septal defect, double outlet right ventricle, double inlet left ventricle, transposition of the great arteries, interrupted aortic arch and others.

Chiari network
Fenestrated remnant of the right valve of the sinus venosus resulting from incomplete regression of this structure during embryogenesis and first described in 1897 (Chiari H. Ueber Netzbildungen im rechten Vorhof. *Beitr Pathol Anat* 1897, 22, 1–10). The prevalence is 2% in autopsy and echocardiography studies. It presents with coarse right atrial reticula connected to the Eustachian and Thebesian valves and attached to the crista terminalis. It may be associated with patent foramen ovale and interatrial septal aneurysm.

cleft AV valve
see atrioventricular valve; *see also* atrial septal defect. *see also* ostium primum ASD.

coarctation of the aorta
A stenosis of the proximal descending aorta varying in anatomy, physiology and clinical presentation. It may present with discrete or long-segment stenosis, is frequently associated with hypoplasia of the aortic arch and bicuspid aortic valve and may be part of a Shone complex.

common (as in: AV valve, atrium, ventricle, etc.)
Implies bilateral structures with absent septation. Contrasts with "single", which implies absence of corresponding contralateral structure. *see also* single.

common atrium
Large atrium characterized by a nonrestrictive communication between the bilateral atria due to the absence of most of the atrial septum. Frequently associated with complex congenital heart disease (isomerism, atrioventricular septal defect, etc.). *see also* single (atrium).

common arterial trunk
see truncus arteriosus.

complete transposition of the great arteries
syn. classic transposition; d-transposition; d-TGA; atrioventricular concordance with ventriculo-arterial discordance. An anomaly wherein the aorta arises from the right ventricle and the pulmonary artery arises from the left ventricle. The right ventricle supports the systemic circulation.

concordant atrioventricular connections
Appropriate connection of morphologic right atrium to morphologic right ventricle and of morphologic left atrium to morphologic left ventricle. *syn.* atrioventricular concordance.

concordant ventriculo-arterial connections
Appropriate origin of pulmonary trunk from morphologic right ventricle and of aorta from morphologic left ventricle. *syn.* ventriculo-arterial concordance.

conduit
A structure that connects non-adjacent parts of the cardiovascular system, allowing blood to flow between them. Often fashioned from prosthetic material. May include a valve.

congenital coronary arteriovenous fi stula (CCAVF)
A direct communication between a coronary artery and cardiac chamber, great artery or vena cava, bypassing the coronary capillary network.

congenital heart disease (CHD)
Anomalies of the heart originating in fetal life. Their expression may, however, be delayed beyond the neonatal period, and may change with time as further postnatal physiologic and anatomic changes occur.

congenitally corrected transposition of the great arteries
syn. cc-TGA; l-transposition; l-TGA; atrioventricular discordance with ventriculo-arterial discordance; double discordance. An anomaly wherein the aorta arises from the right ventricle and the pulmonary artery from the left ventricle, and, in addition, the atrioventricular connection is discordant such that the right atrium connects to the left ventricle and the left atrium connects to the right ventricle. There are usually associated anomalies, the most common being ventricular septal defect, pulmonic stenosis, and/or a hypoplastic ventricle. The right ventricle supports the systemic circulation.

congenital pericardial defect
A defect in the pericardium due to defective formation of the pleuro-pericardial membrane of the septum transversum. The spectrum of pericardial deficiency is wide. It may be partial or total. Its clinical diagnosis is diffi cult. Left-sided defects are more common. Total absence of the pericardium may be associated with other defects such as bronchogenic cyst, pulmonary sequestration, hypoplastic lung, and other congenital heart diseases.

connection
Anatomic link between two structures (e.g. veno-atrial, atrioventricular, ventriculo-arterial).

cono-truncal abnormality
Neural crest cell migration is crucial for cono-truncal septation and the development of both the pulmonary and aortic outflow tracts. If neural crest cell migration fails, cono-truncal abnormalities occur. The most common cono-truncal anomalies are truncus arteriosus and interrupted aortic arch. Other defects may include tetralogy of Fallot, pulmonary atresia with ventricular septal defect, absent pulmonary valve or d-malposition of the great arteries with double outlet right ventricle, single ventricle or tricuspid atresia. Abnormal neural crest migration may also be associated with complex clinical entities, such as CATCH 22.

conus
see infundibulum.

cor triatriatum sinister
A membrane divides the left atrium into an accessory pulmonary venous chamber and a left atrial chamber contiguous with the mitral valve. The pulmonary veins enter the accessory chamber. The connection between the accessory chamber and the true left atrium varies in size and may produce pulmonary venous obstruction.

cor triatriatum dexter
Abnormal septation of the right atrium due to failure of regression of the right valve of the sinus venosus. This yields a smooth-walled posteromedial "sinus" chamber (embryologic origin of the sinus venosus) that receives the venae cavae and (usually) the coronary sinus, and a trabeculated anterolateral "atrial" chamber (embryologic origin of the primitive right atrium) that includes the right atrial appendage and is related to the tricuspid valve. Usually, there is free communication between these two compartments, but variable obstruction to systemic venous flow from the "sinus" chamber to the "atrial" chamber may occur and may be associated with underdevelopment of downstream right heart structures (e.g. hypoplastic tricuspid valve, tricuspid atresia, pulmonary stenosis or pulmonary atresia). A patent foramen ovale or an atrial septal defect are often present in relation to the posteromedial chamber.
    When there is more extensive resorption of the right valve of the sinus venosus, remnants form the Eustachian valve related to the inferior vena cava, the Thebesian valve related to the coronary sinus, and the crista terminalis. Chiari network describes right atrial reticula, which are extensively fenestrated remnants of the right sinus venosus valve. *see* sinus venosus.

criss-cross heart
syn. criss-cross atrioventricular connection. A rotational abnormality of the ventricular mass around its long axis resulting in relationships of the ventricular chambers not anticipated from the given atrioventricular connections. If the rotated ventricles are in a markedly supero-inferior relationship, the heart may

also be described as a supero-inferior or upstairs-downstairs heart. There may be ventriculo-arterial concordance or discordance.

crista supraventricularis
A saddle-shaped muscular crest in the right ventricular outflow tract intervening between the tricuspid valve and the pulmonary valve, consisting of septal and parietal components, which demarcates the junction between the outlet septum and the pulmonary infundibulum. Occasionally, but less accurately termed crista ventricularis.

crista terminalis
A vestigial remnant of the right valve of the sinus venosus located at the junction of the trabeculated right atrial appendage and the smooth-walled "sinus" component of the right atrium component receiving the inferior vena cava, the superior vena cava, and the coronary sinus. A feature of right atrial internal anatomy. *syn.* terminal crest.

crista ventricularis
see crista supraventricularis.

cyanosis
A bluish discoloration due to the presence of an increased quantity of desaturated hemoglobin in tissues. In congenital heart disease, cyanosis is generally due to right-to-left shunting through congenital cardiac defects, bypassing the pulmonary alveoli, or due to acquired intrapulmonary shunts (central cyanosis). Cyanosis can also occur due to increased peripheral extraction due, for instance, to critically reduced cutaneous flow (peripheral cyanosis).

Dacron®
A synthetic material often used to fashion conduits and other prosthetic devices for the surgical palliation or repair of congenital heart disease.

Damus-Kaye-Stansel operation
A procedure reserved for patients with abnormal ventriculo-arterial connections who are not suitable for an arterial switch operation (e.g. TGA and non-suitable coronary patterns, DORV with severe subaortic stenosis, systemic ventricular outflow tract obstruction in hearts with a univentricular AV connection). The operation involves anastomosis of the proximal end of the transected main pulmonary artery in an end-to-side fashion to the ascending aorta to provide blood flow from the systemic ventricle to the aorta; coronary arteries are not translocated and are perfused in a retrograde fashion. The aortic orifice and a VSD (if present) are closed with a patch. A conduit between the right ventricle and the distal pulmonary artery provides venous blood to the lungs. The procedure was described in 1975. (Damus PS. Correspondence. *Annals of Thoracic Surgery* 1975, **20**, 724–725.) (Kaye MP. Anatomic correction of transposition of the great arteries. *Mayo Clinic Proceedings* 1975, **50**, 638–640.)

(Stansel HC Jr. A new operation for d-loop transposition of the great vessels. *Annals of Thoracic Surgery* 1975, **19**, 565–567.)

David operation
A surgical procedure for ascending aortic aneurysm, involving replacement of the ascending aorta with a synthetic tube and remodeling of the aortic root so the preserved aortic valve is no longer regurgitant (David TE, Feindel CM. An aortic valve sparing operation for patients with aortic incompetence and aneurysm of the ascending aorta. *Journal of Thoracic and Cardiovascular Surgery* 1992, **103**, 617–621.)

dextrocardia
Cardiac apex directed to the right of the midline. *see* cardiac position.

dextroposition
Rightward shift of the heart. *see* cardiac position.

dextroversion
An old term for dextrocardia. *see* cardiac position.

differential hypoxemia; differential cyanosis
A difference in the degree of hypoxemia/cyanosis in different extremities as a result of the site of a right-to-left shunt. The most common situation is of greater hypoxemia/cyanosis in feet and sometimes left hand, as compared to right hand and head, in a patient with an Eisenmenger PDA.

DiGeorge syndrome
An autosomal dominant syndrome now known to be part of "CATCH 22". As originally described, it consisted of infantile hypocalcemia, immunodeficiency due to thymic hypoplasia, and a cono-truncal cardiac abnormality. *see also* CATCH 22.

discordant atrioventricular connections
Anomalous connection of atria and ventricles such that the morphologic right atrium connects via a mitral valve to a morphologic left ventricle, while the morphologic left atrium connects via a tricuspid valve to a morphologic right ventricle.

discordant ventriculo-arterial connections
Anomalous connection of the great arteries and ventricles such that the pulmonary trunk arises from the left ventricle and the aorta arises from the right ventricle.

diverticulum of Kommerell
Enlarged origin of the left subclavian artery associated with right aortic arch. Its diameter may be equal to that of the descending aorta and tapers to the left

subclavian diameter. It is found at the origin of the aberrant left subclavian artery, the fourth branch off the right aortic arch.

double aortic arch
see aortic arch anomaly.

double-chambered RV
Separation of the right ventricle (RV) into a higher-pressure inflow chamber, and a lower pressure infundibular chamber, the separation usually being produced by hypertrophy of the "septomarginal band". When a VSD is present, it usually communicates with the high pressure RV inflow chamber.

double discordance
see congenitally corrected transposition of the great arteries.

double inlet left ventricle (DILV)
see univentricular connection.

double orifice mitral valve
The mitral valve orifice is partially or completely divided into two parts by a fibrous bridge of tissue. Both orifices enter the left ventricle. Mitral regurgitation and/or mitral stenosis may be present. Aortic coarctation and atrioventricular septal defect are commonly associated defects.

double outlet left ventricle (DOLV)
Both the pulmonary artery and the aorta arise predominantly from the morphologic left ventricle. DOLV is rare, and much less frequent than double outlet right ventricle (DORV).

double outlet right ventricle (DORV)
Both great arteries arise predominantly from the morphologic right ventricle; there is usually no fibrous continuity between the semilunar and the AV valves; a ventricular septal defect is present. When the VSD is in the subaortic position without RV outflow tract obstruction, the physiology simulates a simple VSD. With RV outflow tract obstruction, the physiology simulates tetralogy of Fallot. When the VSD is in the subpulmonary position (the Taussig-Bing anomaly), the physiology simulates complete transposition of the great arteries with VSD. *see also* Taussig-Bing anomaly.

double switch procedure
An operation used in patients with l-transposition of the great arteries (l-TGA; congenitally corrected transposition of the great arteries; cc-TGA) and also in patients who have had a prior Mustard or Senning atrial switch operation for complete transposition of the great arteries (d-TGA). It leads to anatomic correction of the ventricle to great artery relationships such that the left ventricle

supports the systemic circulation. It includes an arterial switch procedure (*see* Jatene operation) in all cases, as well as an atrial switch procedure (Mustard or Senning) in the case of l-TGA, or reversal of the previously done Mustard or Senning procedure in the case of d-TGA.

doubly-committed VSD
see ventricular septal defect.

Down syndrome
The most common malformation caused by trisomy 21. Most of the patients (95%) have complete trisomy of chromosome 21; some have translocation or mosaic forms. The phenotype is diagnostic (short stature, characteristic facial appearance, mental retardation, brachydactyly, atlanto-axial instability, thyroid and white blood cell disorders). Congenital heart defects are frequent, atrioventricular septal defect and ventricular septal defect being the most common. Mitral valve prolapse and aortic regurgitation may be present. Down syndrome patients are prone to earlier and more severe pulmonary vascular disease than might otherwise be expected as a consequence of the lesions identified.

dural ectasia
Expansion of the dural sac in the lumbo-sacral area, seen on CT or MRI. It is one of the criteria used to confirm the diagnosis of Marfan syndrome. (Pyeritz RE, *et al.* Dural ectasia is a common feature of the Marfan syndrome *American Journal of Human Genetics* 1988, **43**, 726–732.) (Fattori R, *et al.* Importance of dural ectasia in phenotypic assessment of Marfan's syndrome. *Lancet* 1999, **354**, 910–913.)

Ebstein anomaly
An anomaly of the tricuspid valve in which the basal attachments of both the septal and the posterior valve leaflets are displaced apically within the right ventricle. Apical displacement of the septal tricuspid leaflet of >8 mm/M2 is diagnostic (the extent of apical displacement should be indexed to body surface area). Abnormal structure of all three leaflets is seen, with the anterior leaflet typically large with abnormal attachments to the right ventricular wall. The pathologic and clinical spectrum is broad and includes not only valve abnormalities but also myocardial structural changes in both ventricles. Tricuspid regurgitation is common, tricuspid stenosis occurs occasionally, and right-to-left shunting through a patent foramen ovale or atrial septal defect is a regular but not invariable concomitant. Other congenital lesions are often associated, such as VSD, pulmonary stenosis, and/or accessory conduction pathways.

Ehlers-Danlos syndrome (EDS)
A group of heritable disorders of connective tissue, (specifically, abnormalities of collagen). Hyperextensibility of the joints and hyperelasticity and fragility of the skin are common to all forms; patients bruise easily.

- Ehlers-Danlos types I, II and III, which demonstrate autosomal dominant inheritance, are the commonest forms, each representing about 30% of cases. The cardiovascular abnormalities are generally mild, consisting of mitral and tricuspid valve prolapse. Dilatation of major arteries, including the aorta, may occur. Aortic rupture is seen rarely in type I, but not in types II and III.
- Ehlers-Danlos syndrome type IV is also autosomal dominant, but frequently appears de novo. This is the "arterial" form, presenting with aortic dilatation and rupture of medium and large arteries spontaneously or after trauma. It is due to an abnormality of type III procollagen, and comprises about 10% of cases of Ehlers-Danlos syndrome.
- There are 6 other rare types of Ehlers-Danlos syndrome.

Eisenmenger syndrome
An extreme form of pulmonary vascular obstructive disease arising as a consequence of pre-existing systemic to pulmonary shunt, wherein pulmonary vascular resistance rises such that pulmonary pressures are at or near systemic levels and there is reversed (right-to-left) or bidirectional shunting at great vessel, ventricular, and/or atrial levels. *see also* Heath-Edwards classifi cation. *see also* pulmonary hypertension.

Ellis-van Creveld syndrome
An autosomal recessive syndrome in which common atrium, primum ASD and partial AV septal defect are the most common cardiac lesions.

endocardial cushion defect
see atrioventricular septal defect. The term endocardial cushion defect has fallen into disuse because it implies an outdated concept of the morphogenesis of the atrioventricular septum.

erythrocytosis
Increase in red blood cell concentration secondary to chronic tissue hypoxia, as seen in cyanotic CHD and in chronic pulmonary disease. It results from a hypoxia-induced physiologic response resulting in increased erythropoietin levels, and affects only the red cell line. It is also called secondary erythrocytosis. The term "polycythemia" is inaccurate in this context, since other blood cell lines are not affected. *see also* polycythemia vera. Erythrocytosis may cause hyperviscosity symptoms. *see also* hyperviscosity.

Eustachian valve
A remnant of the right valve of the sinus venosus guarding the entrance of the inferior vena cava to the right atrium.

extracardiac Fontan
see Fontan procedure.

fenestration
An opening, or "window" (usually small) between two structures, which may be spontaneous, traumatic, or created surgically.

fibrillin
Fibrillin is a large glycoprotein, closely involved with collagen in the structure of connective tissue. Mutations in the fibrillin gene on chromosome 15 are responsible for all manifestations of Marfan syndrome. *see also* Marfan syndrome.

Fontan procedure (operation)
A palliative operation for patients with a univentricular circulation, involving diversion of the systemic venous return to the pulmonary artery, usually without the interposition of a subpulmonary ventricle. There are many variations, all leading to normalization of systemic oxygen saturation and elimination of volume overload of the functioning ventricle.

- classic Fontan. Originally, a valved conduit between the right atrium and the pulmonary artery (Fontan F, Baudet E. Surgical repair of tricuspid atresia. *Thorax* 1971, **26**, 240–248.) Subsequently changed to a direct anastomosis between right atrium (RA) and pulmonary artery (PA).
- extracardiac Fontan. Inferior vena cava (IVC) blood is directed to the pulmonary artery via an extracardiac conduit. The superior vena cava (SVC) is anastomosed to the PA as in the bidirectional Glenn shunt.
- fenestrated Fontan. Surgical creation of an ASD in the atrial patch or baffle to provide an escape valve, allowing right-to-left shunting to reduce pressure in the systemic venous circuit, at the expense of systemic hypoxemia.
- lateral tunnel. *see* total cavopulmonary connection (TCPC).
- RA-RV Fontan. Conduit (often valved) between right atrium (RA) and right ventricle (RV). Also known as the Björk modification. (Björk VO, *et al.* Right atrial-ventricular anastomosis for correction of tricuspid atresia. *Journal of Thoracic and Cardiovascular Surgery* 1979, **77**, 452–458.)
- total cavopulmonary connection (TCPC). IVC flow is directed by a baffle within the RA into the lower portion of the divided SVC or the right atrial appendage, which is connected to the pulmonary artery. The upper part of the SVC is connected to the superior aspect of the pulmonary artery as in the bidirectional Glenn procedure. The majority of the RA is excluded from the systemic venous circuit. *syn.* lateral tunnel Fontan.

Gerbode defect
An unusual variant of atrioventricular septal defect, wherein the defect is in the superior portion of the atrioventricular septum above the insertion of the septal leaflet of the tricuspid valve, resulting in a direct communication and shunt between the left ventricle and the right atrium. *see also* atrioventricular septum.

Ghent criteria

A set of criteria for the diagnosis of Marfan syndrome, requiring involvement of three organ systems (one system must have "major" involvement), or two organ systems and a positive family history. (DePaepe A, Deitz HC, Devereux RB, *et al.* Revised diagnostic criteria for the Marfan syndrome. *American Journal of Medical Genetics* 1996, **62**, 417–426)

Glenn shunt (operation)

A palliative operation for the purpose of increasing pulmonary blood flow, hence systemic oxygen saturation, in which a direct anastomosis is created between the superior vena cava (SVC) and a pulmonary artery (PA). This procedure does not cause systemic ventricular volume overload.

- classic Glenn. Anastomosis of the SVC to the distal end of the divided right PA with division/ligation of the SVC below the anastomosis. Acquired pulmonary arterio-venous malformations with associated systemic arterial desaturation are a common long-term complication. (Glenn WW. Circulatory bypass of the right side of the heart. IV. Shunt between superior vena cava and distal right pulmonary artery: report of clinical application. *New England Journal of Medicine* 1958, **259**, 117–120.)
- bidirectional Glenn. End-to-side anastomosis of the divided SVC to the undivided PA. (Haller JA Jr, *et al.* Experimental studies in permanent bypass of the right heart. *Surgery* 1966, **59**, 1128–1132.) (Azzolina G, *et al.* Tricuspid atresia: experience in surgical management with a modified cavopulmonary anastomosis. *Thorax* 1972, **27**, 111–115.) (Hopkins RA *et al.* Physiologic rationale for a bi-directional cavopulmonary shunt. A versatile complement to the Fontan principle. *Journal of Thoracic and Cardiovascular Surgery* 1985, **90**, 391–398.)

Gore-Tex®

A synthetic material often used to fashion conduits and other prosthetic devices for the surgical palliation or repair of congenital heart disease.

GUCH

Grown-up congenital heart disease. A term originated by Dr Jane Somerville. *syn.* Adult congenital heart disease.

Heath-Edwards classification

A histopathologic classification useful in assessing the potential for reversibility of pulmonary vascular disease. (Heath D, Edwards JE. The pathology of hypertensive pulmonary vascular disease: A description of six grades of structural changes in the pulmonary arteries with special reference to congenital cardiac septal defects. *Circulation* 1958, **18**, 533–547.)

- Grade I—hypertrophy of the media of small muscular arteries and arterioles.

- Grade II—intimal cellular proliferation in addition to medial hypertrophy.
- Grade III—advanced medial thickening with hypertrophy and hyperplasia including progressive intimal proliferation and concentric fibrosis. This results in obliteration of arterioles and small arteries.
- Grade IV—"plexiform lesions" of the muscular pulmonary arteries and arterioles with a plexiform network of capillary-like channels within a dilated segment.
- Grade V—complex plexiform, angiomatous and cavernous lesions and hyalinization of intimal fi brosis.
- Grade VI—necrotizing arteritis.

hemi-Fontan
The first part of a "staged Fontan", sometimes chosen to reduce the morbidity and mortality that might be associated with performing the complete Fontan at one operation. The hemi-Fontan includes a bidirectional cavopulmonary anastomosis and obliteration of central shunts. The second step to complete the Fontan procedure may be performed at a later time.

hemi-truncus
An anomalous pulmonary artery branch to one lung arising from the ascending aorta in the presence of a main pulmonary artery arising normally from the right ventricle and supplying the other lung.

heterograft
Transplanted tissue or organ from a different species.

heterotaxy
Abnormal arrangement (*taxo* in Greek) of viscera that differs from the arrangement seen in either situs solitus or situs inversus. Often described as "visceral heterotaxy".

heterotopic
Located in an anatomically abnormal site, often in reference to transplantation of an organ.

Holt-Oram syndrome
Autosomal dominant syndrome consisting of radial abnormalities of the forearm and hand associated with secundum ASD (most common), VSD, or, rarely, other cardiac malformations. (Holt M, Oram S. Familial heart disease with skeletal manifestations. *British Heart Journal* 1960, **22**, 236–242.) The gene for this syndrome is on 12q2. (Basson CT, *et al.* The clinical and genetic spectrum of the Holt-Oram syndrome [heart-hand syndrome] *New England Journal of Medicine* 1994, **330**, 885–891.)

homograft
Transplanted tissue or organ from another individual of the same species.

Hunter syndrome

A genetic syndrome due to a deficiency of the enzyme iduronate sulfate (muco-polysaccharidase) with X-linked recessive inheritance. Clinical spectrum is wide. Patients present with skeletal changes, mental retardation, arterial hypertension and involvement of atrioventricular and semilunar valves resulting in valve regurgitation.

Hurler syndrome

A genetic syndrome due to a deficiency of the enzyme a-L-iduronidase (muco-polysaccharidase) with autosomal recessive inheritance. Phenotype presents with a wide spectrum including severe skeletal abnormalities, corneal clouding, hepatosplenomegaly, mental retardation and mitral valve stenosis.

hyperviscosity

An excessive increase in viscosity of blood, as may occur secondary to erythrocytosis in patients with cyanotic congenital heart disease. Hyperviscosity symptoms include: headache; impaired alertness, depressed mentation or a sense of distance; visual disturbances (blurred vision, double vision, amaurosis fugax); paresthesiae of fingers, toes or lips; tinnitus; fatigue, lassitude; myalgias (including chest, abdominal muscles), and muscle weakness. (Perloff JK, *et al.* Adults with cyanotic congenital heart disease: hematologic management. *Annals of Internal Medicine* 1988, **109**, 406–413.) Restless legs or a sensation of cold legs may reflect hyperviscosity (observation of Dr E. Oechslin). As the symptoms are non-specific, their relation to hyperviscosity is supported if they are alleviated by phlebotomy. Iron deficiency and dehydration worsen hyperviscosity and must be avoided, or treated if present.

hypoplastic left heart syndrome

A heterogeneous syndrome with a wide variety and severity of manifestations involving hypoplasia, stenosis, or atresia at different levels of the left heart including the aorta, aortic valve, left ventricular outflow tract, left ventricular body, mitral valve and left atrium.

Ilbawi procedure (operation)

An operation for congenitally corrected transposition of the great arteries with VSD and pulmonary stenosis, wherein a communication is established between the left ventricle (LV) and the aorta via the VSD using a baffle within the right ventricle (RV). The RV is connected to the pulmonary artery using a valved conduit. An atrial switch procedure is done. The LV then supports the systemic circulation. (Ilbawi MN, *et al.* An alternative approach to the surgical management of physiologically corrected transposition with ventricular septal defect and pulmonary stenosis or atresia. *Journal of Thoracic and Cardiovascular Surgery* 1990, **100**, 410–415.)

infracristal
Located below the crista supraventricularis in the right ventricular outflow tract. *see* crista supraventricularis.

infundibular, infundibulum
(Pertaining to) a ventricular-great arterial connecting segment. Normally subpulmonary, but can be sub-aortic, and may be bilateral or absent. Bilateral infundibulum may be seen in patients with TGA/VSD/pulmonary stenosis (PS), DORV with VSD/PS, and anatomically corrected malposition. *syn.* conus.

inlet VSD
see ventricular septal defect.

interrupted aortic arch
see aortic arch anomaly.

interrupted inferior vena cava
The inferior vena cava is interrupted below the hepatic veins with subsequent systemic venous drainage via the azygos vein to the superior vena cava. The hepatic veins enter the right atrium directly. This anomaly is frequently associated with complex congenital heart disease, particularly left-isomerism.

ISACCD
International Society for Adult Congenital Cardiac Disease. For information link through http://www.isaccd.org

isolation of arch vessels
see aortic arch anomalies.

isomerism
Paired, mirror image sets of normally single or non-identical organ systems (atria, lungs, and viscera), often associated with other abnormalities.

- right isomerism. *syn.* asplenia syndrome. Congenital syndrome consisting of paired morphologically right structures: absence of spleen, bilateral right bronchi, bilateral tri-lobed (right) lungs, two morphologic right atria, and multiple anomalies of systemic and pulmonary venous connections and other complex cardiac and non-cardiac anomalies.
- left isomerism. *syn.* polysplenia syndrome. A congenital syndrome consisting of paired, morphologically left structures: multiple bilateral spleens, bilateral left bronchi, bilateral bilobed (left) lungs, midline liver, two morphologic left atria, and complex congenital heart disease and other associated non-cardiac malformations.

Jatene procedure (operation)

syn. arterial switch procedure. An operation used in complete transposition of the great arteries, involving removal of the aorta from its attachment to the right ventricle, and of the pulmonary artery from the left ventricle, and the reattachment of the great arteries to the contralateral ventricles, with reimplantation of the coronary arteries into the neo-aorta. As a consequence, the left ventricle supports the systemic circulation. (Jatene AD, *et al.* Anatomic correction of transposition of the great vessels. *Journal of Thoracic and Cardiovascular Surgery* 1976, **72**, 364–370.) *see also* Lecompte manoeuvre.

juxtaposition of atrial appendages

A rare anomaly seen in patients with transposition of the great arteries and other complex congenital heart defects (dextrocardia, tricuspid atresia, etc.), wherein the atrial appendages are situated side by side. The right atrial appendage passes immediately behind the transposed main pulmonary artery in patients with leftward juxtaposition of atrial appendages.

Kartagener syndrome

Autosomal recessive syndrome consisting of situs inversus totalis, dextrocardia and defect of ciliary motility leading to sinusitis, bronchiectasis and sperm immobility. (Kartegener M. Zur Pathogenese der Bronchiektasien: Bronchiektasien bei Situs viscerum inversus. *Beitr Klink Tuberkul* 1933, **28**, 231–234.) (Kartagener M, *et al.* Bronchiectasis with situs inversus. *Archives of Pediatrics* 1962, **79**, 193–196.) (Miller RD *et al.* Kartagener's syndrome. *Chest* 1972, **62**, 130–136.)

Kommerell

see diverticulum of Kommerell.

Konno procedure (operation)

Repair of tunnel-like subvalvar LVOTO by aorto-ventriculoplasty. The operation involves enlargement of the left ventricular outflow tract by inserting a patch in the ventricular septum, as well as aortic valve replacement and enlargement of the aortic annulus and ascending aorta. (Konno S, *et al.* A new method for prosthetic valve replacement in congenital aortic stenosis associated with hypoplasia of the aortic valve ring. *Journal of Thoracic and Cardiovascular Surgery* 1975, **70**, 909–917.). In severe forms of LVOTO, a prostheticvalve-containing conduit may be inserted between the left ventricular apex and descending aorta. (Didonato RM, *et al.* Left ventricular-aortic conduits in paediatric patients. *Journal of Thoracic and Cardiovascular Surgery* 1984, **88**, 82–91.) (Frommelt PC, *et al.* Natural history of apical left ventricular to aortic conduits in paediatric patients. *Circulation* 1991, **84** (Suppl III), 213–218.)

Lecompte manoeuvre
The pulmonary artery is brought anterior to the aorta during an arterial switch procedure in patients with d-transposition of the great arteries. *see also* Jatene procedure.

LEOPARD syndrome
This autosomal dominant condition includes Lentigines, EKG abnormalities, Ocular hypertelorism, Pulmonary stenosis, Abnormal genitalia, Retardation of growth, and Deafness. Rarely, cardiomyopathy or complex congenital heart disease may be present.

levocardia
Leftward-oriented cardiac apex (normal). *see* cardiac position.

levoposition
Leftward shift of the heart. *see* cardiac position.

ligamentum arteriosum
A normal fibrous structure that is the residuum of the ductus arteriosus after its spontaneous closure.

long-QT syndrome
Abnormal prolongation of QT-duration with subsequent risk for torsade de pointes, syncope and sudden cardiac death. It may be congenital or acquired (medications such as antiarrhythmics, antihistamines, some antibiotics; electrolyte disturbances such as hypocalcemia, hypomagnesemia, hypokalemia; hypothyroidism; and other factors.). QT-interval must be adjusted to heart rate.

looping
Bending of the primitive heart tube (normally to the right, dextro, d-) that determines the atrioventricular relationship.

• d-loop. Morphologic right ventricle lies to the right of the morphologic left ventricle (normal rightward bend).
• l-loop. Morphologic right ventricle lies to the left of the morphologic left ventricle (leftward bend).

Lutembacher syndrome
Atrial septal defect associated with mitral valve stenosis. The mitral valve stenosis is usually acquired (rheumatic).

LVOTO
Left ventricular outflow tract obstruction.

maladie de Roger
Eponymous designation for a small restrictive ventricular septal defect that is not associated with significant left ventricular volume overload or elevated pulmonary artery pressure. There is a loud VSD murmur due to the high velocity turbulent left-to-right shunt across the defect.

malposition
An abnormality of cardiac position. *see* cardiac position.

MAPCA
Major aorto-pulmonary collateral artery. A large abnormal arterial vessel arising from the aorta, connecting to a pulmonary artery (usually in the pulmonary hilum) and providing blood supply to the lungs. Found in complex pulmonary atresia and other complex CHD associated with severe reduction or absence of antegrade pulmonary blood flow from the ventricle(s).

Marfan syndrome
A connective tissue disorder with autosomal dominant inheritance caused by a defect in the fibrillin gene on chromosome 15. The phenotypic expression varies. Patients may have tall stature, abnormal body proportions, ocular abnormalities, dural ectasia, protrusio acetabulae, and present with skeletal and cardiovascular abnormalities. Mitral valve prolapse with mitral regurgitation, ascending aortic dilatation/aneurysm with subsequent aortic regurgitation, and aortic dissection are the most common cardiovascular abnormalities. *see also* Ghent criteria.

mesocardia
Cardiac apex directed to mid-chest. *see* cardiac position.

mesoposition
Shift of the heart toward the midline. *see* cardiac position.

mitral arcade
Chordae of the mitral valve are shortened or absent and the thickened mitral valve leaflets insert directly into the papillary muscle ("hammock valve"). Mitral valve excursion is limited and results in mitral stenosis.

moderator band
A prominent muscular structure traversing the right ventricle from the base of the anterior papillary muscle to the septum near the apex.

muscular VSD
see ventricular septal defect.

Mustard procedure (operation)
An operation for complete transposition of the great arteries, in which venous return is directed to the contralateral ventricle by means of an atrial baffle made from autologous pericardial tissue or (rarely) synthetic material, after resection of most of the atrial septum. As a consequence, the right ventricle supports the systemic circulation. A type of "atrial switch" operation (*see also* Senning procedure, atrial switch procedure, double switch procedure). (Mustard WT. Successful two-stage correction of transposition of the great vessels. *Surgery* 1964, **55**, 469–472.)

national referral center
see supraregional referral center (SRRC).

nonrestrictive VSD
see ventricular septal defect.

Noonan syndrome
An autosomal dominant syndrome phenotypically somewhat similar to Turner syndrome, with a normal chromosomal complement, due to an abnormality in chromosome 12q. It is associated with congenital cardiac anomalies, especially dysplastic pulmonic valve stenosis, pulmonary artery stenosis, ASD, tetralogy of Fallot, or hypertrophic cardiomyopathy. Congenital lymphedema is a common associated anomaly that may be unrecognized. (Noonan JA, Ehmke DA. Associated non-cardiac malformations in children with congenital heart disease. *Midwest Society for Pediatric Research* 1963, **63**, 468.)

Norwood procedure
A multistage operation for hypoplastic left heart syndrome. A systemic to pulmonary arterial shunt is created, followed by a staged Fontan-type operation (usually via a hemi-Fontan procedure) resulting in single ventricle physiology. The morphologic right ventricle supports the systemic circulation.

orthotopic
Located in an anatomically normal recipient site, often in reference to transplantation of an organ.

ostium primum ASD
see atrial septal defect.

outlet VSD
see ventricular septal defect.

over-and-under ventricles
see supero-inferior heart.

overriding valve
An AV valve that empties into both ventricles or a semilunar valve that originates from both ventricles.

palliation, palliative operation
A procedure carried out for the purpose of relieving symptoms or ameliorating some of the adverse effects of an anomaly, which does not address the fundamental anatomic/physiologic disturbance. Contrasts with "repair" or "reparative operation".

PAPVC
Partial anomalous pulmonary venous connection. *see* anomalous pulmonary venous connection.

parachute mitral valve
A mitral valve abnormality in which all chordae tendineae of the mitral valve, which may be shortened and thickened, insert in a single, abnormal papillary muscle, usually causing mitral stenosis. The parachute mitral valve may be part of the Shone complex. *see also* Shone complex.

partial AV septal defect
see atrioventricular septal defect

patent ductus arteriosus (PDA)
A ductus that fails to undergo normal closure in the early postnatal period. *syn:* persistently patent ductus arteriosus, persistent arterial duct.

patent foramen ovale (PFO)
Failure of anatomic fusion of the valve of the foramen ovale with the limbus of the fossa ovalis that normally occurs when left atrial pressure exceeds right atrial pressure after birth. There is no structural deficiency of tissue of the atrial septum. The foramen is functionally closed as long as left atrial pressure exceeds right atrial pressure, but can reopen if right atrial pressure rises. Patent foramen ovale is found in up to 35% of the adult population in pathological studies. The lower and variable prevalence reported in clinical series depends on the techniques used to find it. *syn:* probe-patent foramen ovale, PFO.

pentalogy of Fallot
Tetralogy of Fallot with, in addition, an ASD or PFO. *see* tetralogy of Fallot.

perimembranous VSD
see ventricular septal defect.

persistent left superior vena cava (LSVC)
Persistence of the left anterior cardinal vein (which normally obliterates during embryogenesis) results in persistent left superior vena cava. LSVC drains via the coronary sinus to the right atrium in more than 90% of patients. Rarely, it may directly drain to the left atrium in association with other congenital heart defects (e.g. isomerism). Its prevalence is up to 0.5% in the general population, and higher in patients with congenital heart disease.

PFO
see patent foramen ovale.

phlebotomy
A palliative procedure involving withdrawal of whole blood (usually in up to 500 mL increments) which may be offered to patients with cyanotic CHD and secondary erythrocytosis who are experiencing hyperviscosity symptoms. Concomitant volume replacement is usually indicated.

pink tetralogy of Fallot
see tetralogy of Fallot.

polycythemia vera
A neoplastic transformation of all blood cell lines (erythrocyte, leukocyte, and platelet) associated with increased numbers of cells in the peripheral blood. Contrast with secondary erythrocytosis as seen in cyanotic heart disease. *see also* erythrocytosis.

polysplenia syndrome
see isomerism/left isomerism.

Potts shunt
A palliative operation for the purpose of increasing pulmonary blood flow, hence systemic oxygen saturation. The procedure involves creating a small communication between a pulmonary artery and the ipsilateral descending thoracic aorta. Often complicated by the development of pulmonary vascular obstructive disease if too large, or acquired stenosis or atresia of the pulmonary artery if distortion occurs. (Potts WJ, *et al.* Anastomosis of aorta to pulmonary artery: certain types of congenital heart disease. *Journal of the American Medical Association* 1946, **132**, 627–631.)

PPH
Primary pulmonary hypertension. see pulmonary hypertension.

probe-patent foramen ovale
see patent foramen ovale.

protein-losing enteropathy (PLE)
A complication seen following the Fontan operation in which protein is lost via the gut, resulting in ascites, peripheral edema, pleural and pericardial effusions. It is of unknown cause, though exacerbated by high systemic venous pressure. If serum protein and albumin are low, increased alpha-1 antitrypsin in the stool supports the diagnosis of PLE.

protrusio acetabulae
Abnormal displacement of the head of the femur within the acetabulum. A radiological finding useful in the diagnosis of Marfan syndrome.

pseudotruncus arteriosus
Pulmonary atresia with a VSD, biventricular aorta, and pulmonary blood flow provided by systemic to pulmonary collaterals. This anatomic arrangement had previously been called "truncus arteriosus type IV" but is morphogenetically a different lesion from truncus arteriosus. In pseudotruncus, the single vessel arising from the ventricles is an aorta with an aortic valve, not a truncus with a truncal valve, and pulmonary blood flow derives from aorto-pulmonary collateral arteries, not from anomalously connected true pulmonary arteries.

pulmonary artery banding
Surgically created stenosis of the main pulmonary artery performed as a palliative procedure to protect the lungs against high blood flow and pressure when definitive correction of the underlying anomaly is not immediately advisable, e.g. in the setting of a non-restrictive VSD.

pulmonary artery sling
Anomalous origin of the left pulmonary artery from the right pulmonary artery, such that it loops around the trachea. It may be associated with complete cartilaginous rings in the distal trachea and tracheal stenosis. It may occur as an isolated entity or in association with other congenital heart defects.

pulmonary atresia
An imperforate pulmonary valve. When associated with a VSD (variant of tetralogy of Fallot), pulmonary blood flow arises from aorto-pulmonary collaterals, and systemic venous return exits the right heart via the VSD. When associated with intact interventricular septum, pulmonary artery blood supply is via a patent ductus arteriosus, and systemic venous return exits the right heart via an obligatory ASD.

pulmonary hypertension
Raised pulmonary arterial pressure. A common method to define the severity of pulmonary hypertension is the pulmonary/aortic systolic pressure ratio:

Severity	Ratio
mild	0.3, <0.6
moderate	0.6, <0.9
severe	0.9 (Eisenmenger syndrome)

Rashkind procedure
A balloon atrial septostomy performed as a palliative procedure in children with d-TGA. (Rashkind WJ, Miller WW. Creation of an atrial septal defect without thoracotomy: a palliative approach to complete transposition of the great arteries. *Journal of the American Medical Association* 1966, **196**, 991–992.)

Rastelli procedure (operation)
An operation for repair of complete transposition of the great arteries in association with a large VSD and pulmonic stenosis, wherein a communication is established between the left ventricle (LV) and the aorta via the VSD using a baffle within the right ventricle (RV). The RV is connected to the pulmonary artery using a valved conduit, and the LV-PA connection is obliterated. As a consequence, the left ventricle supports the systemic circulation. (Rastelli GC, *et al.* Anatomic correction of transposition of the great arteries with ventricular septal defect and subpulmonary stenosis. *Journal of Thoracic and Cardiovascular Surgery* 1969, **58**, 545–552.)

regional referral center (RRC)
A center for the care of adult patients with CHD, incorporating, at a minimum, cardiology staff with special skills, training, and experience in the management of such patients, and highly skilled echocardiographers.

restrictive right ventricular physiology
Physiologic behavior of the ventricles of some patients, e.g. after repair of tetralogy of Fallot. It may be defined by echocardiography as antegrade pulmonary artery flow in late diastole (a-wave) through all phases of respiration. The pulsed recordings are obtained with the sample volume at the midpoint between the pulmonary valve cusps or remnants and the pulmonary artery bifurcation. (Redington AN, *et al.* Antegrade diastolic pulmonary artery flow as a marker of right ventricular restriction after complete repair of pulmonary atresia with intact ventricular septum and critical pulmonary valve stenosis. *Cardiology in the Young* 1992, **2**, 382–386.)

restrictive VSD
see ventricular septal defect.

right aortic arch
see aortic arch anomalies.

right ventricular dysplasia
see Uhl anomaly.

Ross procedure
A method of aortic valve replacement involving autograft transplantation of the pulmonary valve, annulus and trunk into the aortic position, with reimplantation of the coronary ostia into the neo-aorta. The RVOT is reconstructed with a homograft conduit. (Ross DN. Replacement of aortic valve with a pulmonary autograft. *Lancet* 1967, **2**, 956–958.) (Ross D. Pulmonary valve autotransplantation [the Ross operation]. *Journal of Cardiac Surgery* 1988, **3**, 313–319.)

rubella syndrome
A wide spectrum of malformations caused by rubella infection early in pregnancy, including cataracts, retinopathy, deafness, congenital heart disease, bone lesions, mental retardation, etc. The spectrum of congenital heart lesions is wide and includes pulmonary artery stenosis, patent ductus arteriosus, tetralogy of Fallot, and ventricular septal defect.

Right ventricle (RV) infundibulum
A normal connecting segment between the body of the RV and the pulmonary artery. *syn.* RV conus. *see also* infundibulum.

RVOTO
Right ventricular outflow tract obstruction.

sail sound
An auscultatory finding in some patients with Ebstein anomaly. The S_1 includes mitral valve closure as its first component with a delayed tricuspid component. The abnormally large tricuspid anterior leaflet snapping like a sail catching the wind causes this delayed closure. The sail sound is not an ejection click, although it may simulate one.

scimitar syndrome
A constellation of anomalies including infradiaphragmatic total or partial anomalous pulmonary venous connection of the right lung to the inferior vena cava, often associated with hypoplasia of the right lung and right pulmonary artery (PA). The lower portion of the right lung tends to receive its arterial supply from the abdominal aorta. The name of the syndrome derives from the appearance on PA chest x-ray of the shadow formed by the anomalous pulmonary venous connection, which resembles a Turkish sword, or scimitar.

secondary erythrocytosis
see erythrocytosis. *see also* polycythemia vera.

Senning procedure (operation)
An operation for complete transposition of the great arteries in which venous return is directed to the contralateral ventricle by means of an atrial baffle fashioned in situ by using right atrial wall and interatrial septum. As a consequence, the right ventricle supports the systemic circulation. A type of "atrial switch" operation. *see also* Mustard procedure, atrial switch operation, double switch operation. (Senning A. Surgical correction of transposition of the great vessels. *Surgery* 1959, 45, 966–980.)

Shone complex (syndrome)
An association of multiple levels of left ventricular inflow and outflow obstruction (subvalvar and valvar LVOTO, coarctation of the aorta and mitral stenosis [parachute mitral valve and supramitral ring]). (Shone JD *et al.* The developmental complex of "parachute mitral valve", supravalvular ring of left atrium, subaortic stenosis and coarctation of aorta. *American Journal of Cardiology* 1963, 11, 714–725.)

Shprintzen syndrome
see velo-cardio-facial syndrome. *see* CATCH 22.

shunt
Movement of blood through a congenitally abnormal or surgically created connection and communication between two circuits, at the level of the atria, ventricles, or great vessels. "Shunt" is a physiologic term, in contrast to "connection" which is an anatomic term.

single (as in atrium, ventricle, etc.)
Implies absence of the corresponding contralateral structure. Contrasts with "common", which implies bilateral structures with absent septation. *see also* common.

sinus venosus
An embryologic structure, the anatomic precursor of the inferior vena cava, superior vena cava and coronary sinus and part of the definitive right atrium, which is located external to the primitive right atrium in the early embryologic period (3 to 4 weeks' gestation). The sinus portion of the right atrium receives the inferior vena cava, superior vena cava and coronary sinus. The right and left valves of the sinus venosus separate the sinus venosus from the primitive right atrium, the embryologic precursor of the trabeculated or muscular portion of the right atrium, and includes the right atrial appendage, which in turn communicates with the tricuspid valve. The left valve of the sinus venosus joins the interatrial septum, retrogresses and is absorbed. The right valve of the sinus venosus enlarges and functions to deflect the oxygenated fetal blood coming from the placenta and via the inferior vena cava across the foramen ovale. *see also* cor triatriatum dexter, sinus venosus defect.

sinus venosus defect
A communication located postero-superior (or rarely postero-inferior) to the oval fossa, commonly associated with partial anomalous pulmonary venous connection (most often right pulmonary veins, especially the right upper pulmonary vein in association with a postero-superior defect), which is functionally identical to an atrial septal defect, but properly named a sinus venosus defect because it occurs due to abnormal development of the sinus venosus in relation to the pulmonary veins and is not a defect in the interatrial septum. *see also* atrial septal defect

situs
syn. sidedness. The position of the morphologic right atrium determines the sidedness and is independent of the direction of the cardiac apex, or the positions of the ventricles or the great arteries.

- situs ambiguous. Indeterminate sidedness (in the setting of atrial isomerism).
- situs inversus. Mirror-image sidedness, i.e. opposite of normal. Left-sided morphologic right atrium.
- situs inversus totalis. Total mirror-image sidedness. The position of all lateralized organs is inverted.
- situs solitus. Normal sidedness. Right-sided morphologic right atrium.

stent
Intravascular (intraluminal) prosthesis to scaffold a vessel following transluminal balloon dilatation, for the purpose of maintaining patency.

Sterling Edwards procedure
A palliative operation for transposition of the great arteries in which the atrial septum was resected, repositioned, and sutured to the left of the right pulmonary veins to produce drainage into the right atrium. The procedure produced left-to-right shunt of oxygenated blood directly into the systemic atrium and ventricle and offloaded the pulmonary circulation in patients with complete transposition of the great arteries and high pulmonary flow. (Edwards WS, Bargeron LM, *et al.* Reposition of right pulmonary veins in transposition of the great vessels. *Journal of the American Medical Association* 1964, **188**, 522–523. Edwards WS, Bargeron LM. More effective palliation of the transposition of the great vessels. *Journal of Thoracic and Cardiovascular Surgery* 1965, **19**, 790–795.)

straddling AV valve
see atrioventricular valve.

subpulmonary ventricle
The ventricle that relates most directly to the pulmonary artery.

supero-inferior heart
A term applied to a heart the ventricles of which are in a markedly supero-inferior relationship due to abnormal displacement of the ventricular mass along the horizontal plane of its long axis. Often coexists with criss-cross atrio-ven-tricular relationships. *see also* criss-cross heart. *syn.* over-and-under ventricles; upstairs-downstairs heart.

supracristal
Located above the crista supraventricularis in the right ventricular outflow tract, hence contiguous with the origin of the great arteries. see crista supraventricularis.

supraregional referral center (SRRC)
A "full service" center for providing optimal care of adult patients with CHD comprising specialized resources, the availability of cardiology specialists with specific training and experience in ACHD, the availability of other cardiology sub-specialists and other medical and paramedical personnel with special training/experience in the problems of congenital heart disease, and offering opportunities for training, research and education in the field. *syn.* national referral center.

supravalvar mitral ring
An anomaly found in the left atrium that produces congenital mitral stenosis. *see also* cor triatriatum. *see also* Shone complex.

switch-conversion of transposition
An operation performed in patients with congenitally corrected transposition of the great arteries, or in patients who had previously had a Mustard or Senning procedure for complete transposition of the great arteries, to allow the left ventricle to assume the function of the systemic ventricle. The first stage may involve pulmonary artery banding to induce pulmonary left ventricular hypertrophy. The second stage involves an arterial switch operation in both groups and a Mustard or Senning operation in patients with congenitally corrected transposition, or removal of the Mustard/Senning atrial baffles and reconstruction of an atrial septum in patients with complete TGA. *see also* double switch operation.

systemic AV valve
The atrioventricular valve guarding the inlet to the systemic ventricle.

TAPVC
Total anomalous pulmonary venous connection. *see* anomalous pulmonary venous connection.

TAPVD
Total anomalous pulmonary venous drainage. A term sometimes used to refer to the entity properly called total anomalous pulmonary venous connection. *see* anomalous pulmonary venous connection.

Taussig-Bing anomaly
A form of double outlet right ventricle in which the great arteries arise side-by-side with the aorta to the right of the pulmonary artery and the ventricular septal defect in a subpulmonary position. Since the left ventricle empties across the VSD preferentially into the pulmonary artery, the physiology simulates complete transposition of the great arteries with a VSD.

tetralogy of Fallot
A congenital anomaly, the primary pathophysiologic components of which are obstruction to right ventricular outflow at the infundibular level and a large nonrestrictive VSD. The other two components of the "tetralogy" are an overriding aorta and concentric right ventricular hypertrophy. Valvar RVOTO (pulmonic stenosis) and distal pulmonary artery stenosis are often present. The essential morphogenetic anomaly is malalignment of the infundibular (outlet) septum such that it fails to unite with the trabecular septum (hence the VSD) due to anterior deviation (hence the RVOTO). Lillehei first described the repair in 1955. (Lillehei CW, *et al*. Direct vision intracardiac surgical correction of the tetralogy of Fallot, pentalogy of Fallot, and pulmonary atresia defects; reports of first ten cases. *Annals of Surgery* 1955, **142**, 418–445.)

- pentalogy of Fallot. Tetralogy of Fallot with an associated ASD or PFO.
- pink tetralogy of Fallot. Tetralogy of Fallot presenting with increased pulmonary blood flow and minimal cyanosis because of a lesser degree of RVOTO. *syn.* acyanotic Fallot.

Thebesian valve
A remnant of the right valve of the sinus venosus guarding the opening of the coronary sinus.

total anomalous pulmonary venous connection (drainage, return)
see anomalous pulmonary venous connection/total anomalous pulmonary venous connection.

trabecular VSD
see ventricular septal defect

transannular
Crossing the annulus. In connection with the RVOT in tetralogy of Fallot, the term refers to the pulmonary valve annulus, which often must be enlarged by a transannular patch, with consequent obligatory pulmonary insufficiency. Transannular patching was first described in 1959. (Kirklin JW, *et al*. Surgical treatment for tetralogy of Fallot by open intracardiac repair. *Journal of Thoracic Surgery* 1959, **37**, 22–51.)

transposition of the great arteries (TGA)
see discordant ventriculo-arterial connections and see below

- simple TGA. Discordant connection of the great arteries and ventricles such that the pulmonary trunk arises from the left ventricle and the aorta arises from the right ventricle, without any associated abnormality.
- complex transposition of the great arteries. Discordant connection of the great arteries and ventricles such that the pulmonary trunk arises from the left ventricle and the aorta arises from the right ventricle, with associated abnormalities, most commonly a ventricular septal defect.

tricuspid atresia
A congenital anomaly in which there is no physiologic or gross morphologic connection between the right atrium and right ventricle, and there is an inter-atrial connection allowing mixing of systemic and pulmonary venous return at the atrial level. There is a variable degree of hypoplasia of the right ventricle. The left ventricle and mitral valve are normal.

truncus arteriosus
A single artery (truncus) arises from the base of the heart because of failure of proximal division into the aorta and the pulmonary artery. Thus, both pulmonary and systemic arteries as well as the coronary arteries arise from the common trunk. Truncus arteriosus is divided into two types depending on whether there is a VSD or an intact ventricular septum. *syn.* common arterial trunk.

Turner syndrome
A clinical syndrome due to the 45 XO karyotype in about 50% of cases, with 45XO/45XX mosaicism and other X chromosome abnormalities comprising the remainder. There is a characteristic but variable phenotype, and association with congenital cardiac anomalies, especially post-ductal coarctation of the aorta and other left-sided obstructive lesions, as well as partial anomalous pulmonary venous drainage without ASD. The female phenotype varies with the age of presentation, and is somewhat similar to that of Noonan syndrome.

Uhl anomaly
Congenital malformation consisting of nearly total absence of the right ventricular myocardium, presenting with marked enlargement of both the right ventricle and right atrium and subsequent tricuspid regurgitation. Arrhythmogenic right ventricular cardiomyopathy may be one end of a spectrum and Uhl anomaly the other.

unbalanced AV canal
see ventricular imbalance.

unifocalization
A surgical technique that creates a common trunk for multiple direct aortopulmonary collateral arteries, as part of the surgical management of complex pulmonary atresia.

univentricular connection
Both atria are connected to only one ventricle. The connection is univentricular, but the heart is usually biventricular.

unroofed coronary sinus
An anomaly in which there is a deficiency in the normal separation of the coronary sinus from the left atrium as the coronary sinus passes behind the left atrium (LA) in the AV groove, such that the coronary sinus drains into the LA. A form of absence of the coronary sinus.

upstairs-downstairs heart
see supero-inferior heart.

VACTERL association
Describes a spectrum of defects including vertebral abnormalities, anal atresia, tracheo-esophageal fistula, radial dysplasia, renal abnormalities and congenital heart defects (atrial and ventricular septal defect, tetralogy of Fallot, truncus arteriosus, aortic coarctation, patent ductus arteriosus, etc.).

vascular ring
A wide spectrum of aortic arch anomalies including double aortic arch and other vascular structures that surround the trachea and the esophagus resulting in their compression. The vascular structures may or may not be patent. Vascular rings may be isolated (in 1% to 2% of CHD) or associated with other CHD malformations, such as tetralogy of Fallot. *see* aortic arch anomalies.

velo-cardio-facial syndrome
Syndrome of cleft palate, abnormal facies (square nasal root, long nose with narrow alar base, long face with malar hypoplasia, long philtrum, thickened helix, low set ears), velopharyngeal incompetence and congenital cardiac defects (cono-truncal anomalies, isolated VSD, tetralogy of Fallot). Due to microdeletion at chromosome 22q11. *syn.* Shprintzen syndrome. *see also* CATCH 22.

venous (or pulmonary) AV valve
The AV valve guarding the inlet to the venous, or pulmonary, ventricle.

ventricle repair

- 1-ventricle repair. *see* Fontan operation
- 1.5-ventricle repair (one and one-half ventricle repair). A term used to describe operations for cyanotic congenital heart disease performed when the pulmonary ventricle is insufficiently developed to accept the entire systemic venous return. A bidirectional cavopulmonary connection is constructed to divert superior vena cava flow directly to the lungs, while inferior vena cava flow is directed to the lungs via the functioning but small pulmonary ventricle.

- 2-ventricle repair. A term used to describe operations for cyanotic congenital heart disease with common ventricle wherein functioning systemic and pulmonary ventricles are created by means of surgical septation of the common ventricle.

ventricular imbalance
In the setting of atrioventricular septal defect, ventricular imbalance refers to relative hypoplasia of one or the other of the ventricles in association with small size of the ipsilateral component of the atrioventricular annulus.

ventricular septal defect (VSD)
A defect in the ventricular septum, such that there is direct communication between the two ventricles.

- doubly-committed VSD. A defect in the outlet septum such that there is fibrous continuity between the aortic and pulmonary valves, with the VSD situated directly beneath both semilunar valves.
- inlet VSD. A defect in the lightly trabeculated inlet portion of the muscular interventricular septum, typically seen as part of an atrioventricular septal defect.
- muscular VSD. A defect entirely surrounded by muscular interventricular septum.
- nonrestrictive VSD. A ventricular septal defect of such a size that there is no significant pressure gradient between the ventricles. Hence, the pulmonary artery is exposed to systemic pressure unless there is RVOTO.
- outlet VSD. A defect in the non-trabeculated outlet portion of the muscular interventricular septum, hence above the crista supraventricularis. *syn.* supracristal VSD. Sometimes also described as subpulmonary, subarterial, or doubly committed subarterial VSD.
- perimembranous VSD. A VSD located in the membranous portion of the interventricular septum with variable extension into the contiguous portions of the inlet, trabecular, or outlet portions of the muscular septum, but not involving the atrioventricular septum. *syn.* membranous VSD; infracristal VSD.
- restrictive VSD. A ventricular septal defect of small enough size that there is a pressure gradient between the ventricles, such that the pulmonary ventricle (hence pulmonary vasculature) is protected from the systemic pressure of the contralateral ventricle.
- trabecular VSD. A defect in the heavily trabeculated central or trabecular portion of the muscular interventricular septum. May be multiple.

ventriculo-arterial concordance
see concordant ventriculo-arterial connections.

ventriculo-arterial discordance
see discordant ventriculo-arterial connections.

Waterston shunt

A palliative operation for the purpose of increasing pulmonary blood flow, hence systemic oxygen saturation, which involves creating a small communication between the main pulmonary artery and the ascending aorta. Often complicated by the development of pulmonary vascular obstructive disease if too large. Not uncommonly caused distortion of the pulmonary artery. (Waterston DJ. Treatment of Fallot's tetralogy in children under one year of age. *Rozhl Chir* 1962, **41**, 181–183.)

Williams syndrome

An autosomal dominant syndrome, often arising de novo, associated with an abnormality of elastin, infantile hypercalcemia, mild cognitive impairment and the so-called "cocktail personality", and congenital heart disease, especially supravalvar aortic stenosis and multiple peripheral pulmonary stenoses. (Williams JC, *et al.* Supravalvular aortic stenosis. *Circulation* 1961, **24**, 1311–1318.) (Beuren A, *et al.* Supravalvular aortic stenosis in association with mental retardation and certain facial features. *Circulation* 1962, **26**, 1235–1240.)

Wolff-Parkinson-White (WPW) syndrome

Accessory lateral atrioventricular conduction pathway causing characteristic EKG changes and atrial (and sometimes ventricular) arrhythmias. WPW syndrome may be isolated or associated with congenital heart defects. It is found in up to 25% of patients with Ebstein anomaly. Typically, they have more than one accessory pathway.

Wood unit

A non-standard unit for expressing pulmonary vascular resistance (mmHg/L), named after Paul Wood, the famous British cardiologist. One Wood unit is equivalent to 80 dyn.cm.sec^{-5}.

xenograft

Tissue or organ used for transplant, derived from another species. *syn.* Heterograft.

Z-score, Z-value

A way of expressing a physiologic variable in a form corrected for age and body size. Important in pediatrics. This is the number of standard deviations a measurement departs from mean normal. (Rimoldi HJA, *et al.* A note on the concept of normality and abnormality in quantitation of pathologic findings in congenital heart disease. *Pediatric Clinics of North America* 1963, **10**, 589–591.) (Daubeney PEF, *et al.* Relationship of the dimension of cardiac structures to body size: an echocardiographic study in normal infants and children. *Cardiology in the Young* 1999, **9**, 402–410.)

Index

Printed in Singapore